National Registry Paramedic

Prep Book

2023-2024

- 📓 **Note-Taking Techniques:** Discover various methods for taking effective and organized notes during lectures or while reading textbooks.
- 💬**Critical Thinking Skills:** Develop your ability to analyze, evaluate, and synthesize information to make informed decisions and solve problems.
- ⏰ **Time Blocking and the Pomodoro Technique:** Learn about time management techniques like time blocking and the Pomodoro Technique to enhance productivity
- 🏆 **Stress Relief Strategies:** Overcome exam anxiety with mindfulness, relaxation exercises, and mental resilience techniques.
- ⬛**Practice Makes Perfect:** Explore the importance of practice exams, sample questions, and mock tests, and understand how to analyze your performance to identify areas for improvement.
- ⚫ **Test-Taking Tactics:** Master the art of answering different types of questions, managing your time during the exam, and maintaining focus under pressure.

TABLE OF CONTENT

STUDY GUIDE

Chapter 5: Patient Assessment

The Primary Survey
The Secondary Survey
Special Considerations
Documentation

Chapter 6: Airway and Breathing

Airway Management
Mechanical Ventilation
Respiratory Emergencies
Monitoring and Oxygenation

Chapter 7: Cardiology

Anatomy of the Heart
ECG Interpretation
Cardiac Arrhythmias
Cardiac Emergencies

Chapter 8: Trauma

Trauma Assessment
Trauma Resuscitation
Musculoskeletal Injuries
Head and Spinal Injuries

Chapter 9: Medical Emergencies

Endocrine and Metabolic Disorders
Gastrointestinal Disorders
Neurological Emergencies
Infectious Diseases

Chapter 10: Obstetrics and Pediatrics

Maternal and Fetal Health
Pediatric Assessment
Pediatric Emergencies
Special Considerations for Children

Chapter 11: Operations

EMS Systems
Legal and Ethical Considerations
Infection Control
Disaster Preparedness

Chapter 12: Practice Exams

Sample Questions for Each Chapter
Answer Keys and Explanations

Chapter 13: Final Review and Test-Day Strategies

Preparing for the National Registry Exam
Test-Taking Strategies
Stress Management

Chapter 14: Resources and Additional Study Aids

Online Resources
Recommended Books
Review Courses and Workshops

Chapter 15: Special Populations

Geriatric Patients
Patients with Special Needs
Cultural Competence in EMS
Providing Care in Unique Situations

Chapter 16: Environmental Emergencies

Heat-Related Illnesses
Cold-Related Emergencies
Environmental Toxins and Hazards
Wilderness Medicine

Chapter 17: Advanced Life Support

Advanced Airway Management
Intravenous Access and Medications
Cardiac Arrest Management
Post-Resuscitation Care

Chapter 18: Trauma Systems and Triage

Trauma Centers and Designation
Triage Systems
Mass Casualty Incidents

Before we begin:

You have found yourself in the year 2023-2024 edition of the National Registry Paramedic Prep Book. As you begin your road toward becoming a licensed paramedic, this detailed handbook is intended to serve as a resource that you can always turn to for assistance. This book is intended to support you in accomplishing your goals, whether you are a student getting ready for the National Registry Paramedic Exam, an experienced paramedic looking to refresh your knowledge, or a dedicated educator guiding the future generation of EMS professionals.

The field of emergency medical services, sometimes known as EMS, is one that is both active and tough. In this field, medical professionals are frequently the first people to arrive at the scenes of accidents, trauma, and medical emergencies. In order to offer life-saving care in high-pressure situations, paramedics need to have a strong understanding of human anatomy, physiology, and pharmacology as well as strong critical thinking skills. This requires a significant amount of education and training.

Regarding This Book

This book is more than simply a study guide; it is an all-encompassing resource that covers the range of knowledge and abilities you need in order to flourish in the field of emergency medical services (EMS). You can use the information on these pages to build a strong foundation in emergency medical services (EMS), whether you are studying for the National Registry Paramedic Exam or want to improve your clinical practice. The content has been organized to do so.

The content areas that are tested on the National Registry Paramedic Exam have been mapped out into a sequence of chapters that correspond to the organization of the book. Each chapter digs into a unique topic matter, ranging from cardiac emergencies, trauma, pediatrics, and more to anatomy and physiology. In addition to this, it provides you with useful knowledge on the operations of EMS, legal and ethical issues, and professional growth, all of which are crucial to your success as a paramedic.

The Exam to Become a Paramedic for the National Registry

Obtaining your national certification as a paramedic is a big accomplishment and a critical stage in the progression of your emergency medical services career. The National Registry of Emergency Medical Technicians (NREMT), which is a highly regarded institution, is in charge of ensuring that emergency medical service personnel all throughout the United States are qualified and up to standard. applicants must earn a passing score on the National Registry of Emergency Medical Technicians (NREMT) Paramedic Exam in order to become certified as paramedics. This exam evaluates applicants' knowledge, abilities, and competence to provide advanced life support in prehospital settings.

The National Registry of Emergency Medical Technicians (NREMT) Paramedic Exam is a demanding and extensive test that covers a wide variety of subject areas, such as patient evaluation, airway management, pharmacology, cardiology, trauma, pediatrics, and many more. It is not simply a test of your ability to memorize information; rather, it is a display of your capacity to apply what you have learned in hypothetical situations.

This book is intended to assist you in preparing for the National Registry of Emergency Medical Technicians (NREMT) Paramedic Exam by providing a methodical approach to learning and enhancing your familiarity with fundamental ideas. You will discover detailed explanations, real-world examples, and practice questions that mirror the structure and subject matter of the real exam sprinkled throughout the entirety of the book.

Instructions for Using This Book

This book, the National Registry Paramedic Prep Book, is designed to be a resource that is adaptable and simple to use. The following are some suggestions on how to get the most out of reading this book:

To study in a methodical manner, start with the chapters that correspond to the learning requirements or curriculum you are now following. Read over the offered material, make notes as you go, and get involved with the provided practice questions.

Exercises and Practice Questions You will find exercises and practice questions at the end of each chapter that test your grasp of the material that was presented. Make use of these questions to conduct a self-evaluation and brush up on your knowledge.

Review and Reflect: The book includes a chapter that is devoted to a final review as well as tactics for exam day. You should take advantage of this time to review previously learned material and practice answering test questions in order to improve your overall performance.

You should practice with the practice tests for the National Registry that are offered in Chapter 22 as soon as you are prepared to do so. You will get a feel for the actual examination conditions through these simulated exams, which will also help you evaluate your level of preparedness.

Explore the recommended resources in Chapter 14, which can give you with further help for your studies, and make use of any other study aids that may come in handy. There is a multitude of extra material available to assist your preparation, ranging from recommended books and online refresher courses to internet resources and other reading materials.

Do not skip Chapter 21 if you want a more in-depth comprehension of how the information you learn in this book is utilized in actual emergency medical services (EMS) scenarios. Case Studies and Scenarios. Case studies and hypothetical situations offer essential insights into the process of clinical decision-making.

Conclusions and Suggestions for the Future: Chapter 23 will provide you with direction on what to do once you have successfully completed the NREMT Paramedic Exam. It will also offer advice on how to progress your career and the significance of continuing your professional development.

Certification for Paramedics and the National Registry is Discussed in Chapter 1.

The path to becoming a paramedic is one that is both honorable and difficult to travel. It is a path that needs devotion, education, and a commitment to giving treatment that could potentially save the lives of individuals who are in need. In this chapter, we look into the fundamentals of paramedic certification and the function that the National Registry of Emergency Medical Technicians (NREMT) plays in determining the standards that paramedics in the United States are held to and the expectations that are placed on them. We are going to discuss the relevance of certification, the fundamental duties of a paramedic, and the adventure that you are about to start upon.

Prerequisites for Obtaining a Paramedic Certification

The field of emergency medicine places paramedics in the vanguard of patient care; frequently, they provide the greatest quality of prehospital treatment available. They are prepared to give advanced life support, administer drugs, and make crucial judgments in high-pressure situations thanks to the training they have received. The job of a paramedic is one that is difficult but also gratifying, and earning one's certification in this field is a considerable accomplishment in and of itself. Let's start by discussing the prerequisites and duties linked with the position of paramedic so that we can get a better grasp on the significance of obtaining this certification.

The Value of Accreditation for Businesses

Certification is an official process that acknowledges an individual's skills and level of expertise in a particular area of study or work. Certification is not only a mark of distinction for paramedics; rather, it is necessary from both a moral and a legal standpoint. In order to work as paramedics in the United States, emergency medical services workers need to have the required certification.

There are a variety of factors to consider while deciding whether or not to pursue certification in the field of emergency medical services. The necessity of paramedic certification cannot be overstated, and the following are some of the primary reasons why:

Patient Safety: Ensuring patient safety should always come first when considering a certification program. Individuals who are in life-threatening situations place their trust in the care provided by paramedics. Certification is a means for validating that paramedics have the information, skills, and training necessary to offer the highest level of care to patients. Certification helps ensure that paramedics can give patients with the best possible treatment.

Standardization: Certification plays an important role in helping to standardize the level of care that is offered across a variety of EMS systems and jurisdictions. It makes certain that paramedics meet a standard set of requirements and are ready to deal with the same kinds of situations regardless of the location in which they are employed.

Legal Requirements: To be able to work as a paramedic in many states, one must first earn their paramedic certification. People are not permitted to offer prehospital care if they do not have the appropriate qualification, and if they do so nonetheless, they risk facing legal repercussions.

Certification might have an effect on the insurance coverage and liability protection that are available to EMS companies and providers. As part of the criterion for hiring and continuing employment, qualification requirements for paramedics are frequently imposed by employers.

Certification is an indication of a practitioner's commitment to remaining professionally competent in their industry. It conveys the message that paramedicine is a highly regarded profession that has stringent requirements for training and competency.

Opportunities for Career Advancement Obtaining a certification as a paramedic makes it possible to pursue a variety of career advancement opportunities, such as specialized roles within the EMS system, teaching, research, and leadership positions.

Different Levels of Certification for Paramedics

Certification in the field of emergency medical services (EMS) is more comprehensive than that of paramedics, which is how certification works in the United States. There are several levels of certification for emergency medical services (EMS), beginning with Emergency Medical Responder (EMR) and progressing all the way up to Paramedic. The position of paramedic is considered to be the highest degree of prehospital care; hence, it comes with the most thorough training and the most significant responsibility.

Let's take a more in-depth look at the progression of EMS certification levels, which goes as follows:

The Emergency Medical Responder (EMR) certification is the first step toward a career in emergency medical services (EMS). EMRs receive the training necessary to give fundamental emergency treatment while waiting for more advanced medical personnel, such as EMTs or paramedics, to arrive at the location. Skills in basic life support (BLS) are incorporated into their training.

Emergency Medical Technician (EMT): The scope of practice for EMTs is significantly more extensive than that of EMRs. They have received the necessary training to offer BLS care and are able to give oxygen, perform CPR, and employ procedures for basic airway control. When there is an emergency, it is common for EMTs to be the first EMS providers to arrive at the scene.

The Advanced Emergency Medical Technician (AEMT) level is designed to bridge the gap between the EMT level and the paramedic level. AEMTs receive additional training in areas such as intravenous (IV) therapy and the administration of a select number of drugs. These are only two examples of the expanded scope of their responsibilities.

The highest degree of emergency medical services (EMS) certification is known as the paramedic. The administration of a wide variety of drugs, sophisticated airway management, and complex medical procedures are some of the skills that are covered in the rigorous training that paramedics get in advanced life support (ALS) techniques. They are the primary caregivers for patients who are gravely ill or have been seriously damaged.

To become a paramedic, you must first earn your certification as an emergency medical technician. Before enrolling in paramedic training, many schools require candidates to have completed a certain number of hours of emergency medical technician (EMT) training first. Before moving on to the more advanced skills and knowledge required of paramedics, it is imperative that applicants have this experience under their belts to ensure that they have a solid basic grasp of prehospital care.

Instruction and Learning in Paramedic Work

Training to become a paramedic is challenging and time-consuming since it is designed to teach you the knowledge and skills necessary to offer advanced life support in prehospital settings. Instruction in the classroom and practical training in the field are often both required components of the paramedic curriculum. Let's have a look at some of the most important aspects of paramedic training:

Instruction in the Classroom Students studying to become paramedics spend their time in the classroom delving into a wide variety of subjects, such as anatomy and physiology, pharmacology, cardiology, trauma treatment, pediatrics, and many more. These subjects are necessary for gaining an awareness of the human body, medical conditions, and the interventions that are required to be carried out by paramedics.

Clinical Rotations: Students studying to become paramedics spend a large portion of their time in clinical settings, where they are able to receive hands-on experience in a variety of healthcare settings. Work in hospital emergency departments, surgery rooms, and other areas pertinent to their training are included in this.

Internship in the Field The field internship is an essential component of the education required to become a paramedic. During this phase, students work side-by-side with experienced paramedics in prehospital settings such as ambulances or other locations outside of hospitals. They receive practical experience in assessing patients, providing treatment to those assessments, and making treatment decisions.

Training in Practical Skills The majority of paramedic schools include an emphasis on training students in a variety of practical skills, including intravenous (IV) access, intubation, cardiac monitoring, and the administration of drugs. In order for students to graduate, they need to demonstrate that they are proficient in these skills.

Clinical and Didactic Examinations: All the way through their education, students studying to become paramedics are put through a series of tests, both written and practical, to determine whether or not they have mastered the necessary information and are able to effectively apply it.

Exam for National Registry: The National Registry Exam for Paramedics is the capstone of the education required to become a paramedic. applicants must achieve a passing score on this all-encompassing test in order to become certified as paramedics. This test examines applicants' knowledge, clinical skills, and ability to make decisions.

What Exactly Does a Paramedic Do?

Within the context of the healthcare system, the work that paramedics do is essential. They are experts who have received extensive training and respond to a wide variety of emergencies by administering advanced life support and making decisions that have the potential to make the difference between life and death. The following is a list of some of the most important obligations and duties of a paramedic:

Patient Assessment: Paramedics are trained to perform in-depth patient evaluations in order to determine whether a patient has been hurt or is suffering from a medical condition. They use a methodical approach to collecting information, arranging treatment in priority order, and making important decisions.

Management of the Airway: Establishing and maintaining a patient's airway is one of the most important tasks that a paramedic is expected to perform. Intubation and other forms of advanced airway management are included in this category of procedures.

Pharmacology: Paramedics receive extensive training in the administration of a wide variety of pharmaceuticals, including those used for the management of pain, drugs for the treatment of cardiac disorders, and medications to treat a variety of other medical conditions. They are required to have an in-depth knowledge of the activities of drugs and the potential risks associated with them.

Paramedics are frequently the first people to arrive at the scene of a cardiac emergency and provide care. They have received the essential training to identify arrhythmias, begin cardiopulmonary resuscitation (CPR), and provide defibrillation when it is required.

Trauma Care: Paramedics are highly trained in all aspects of trauma care, including the control of bleeding, the immobilization of the spinal column, as well as the evaluation and treatment of injuries sustained as a consequence of accidents or acts of violence.

treatment for Pediatric Patients: Paramedics are trained to offer treatment for pediatric patients, which calls for a specialized set of abilities and knowledge due to the anatomical and physiological distinctions that exist in children.

Prehospital Care: Prehospital care is provided by paramedics, who work outside of hospitals and provide medical assistance in a range of locations, from the scene of an accident to private homes. They have to be able to adjust quickly and be able to give care even in difficult circumstances.

Communication is essential to the job of a paramedic, and it must be done effectively. In order to guarantee that patients receive the right care, they are required to maintain open lines of communication with patients, members of the patients' families, other medical professionals, and dispatchers.

Documentation: It is the responsibility of the paramedic to document the patient's assessment, as well as the care that was delivered and vital signs. Maintaining continuity of care and complying with regulatory requirements both require accurate recordkeeping.

Legal and Ethical Considerations Paramedics are tasked with navigating a maze of complex legal and ethical concerns, including the duty to report specific conditions or incidents, informed consent, and patient confidentiality.

Learning Never Stops: Because the area of medicine is always undergoing new developments, paramedics are required to participate in continuous education and training in order to ensure that they are always up to date on the most recent evidence-based practices and standards.

You are not just a supplier of medical care, but also an essential link in the chain of survival for a great number of patients if you work as a paramedic. Your actions have the potential to have a substantial influence on the outcomes for those you are serving, which makes your role both a privilege and a duty of a considerable kind.

Getting Ready to Achieve Success

Training to become a paramedic is difficult, and preparation for the National Registry Paramedic Exam is not an exception to this rule. To achieve one's goals, one must be dedicated, willing to put in hard work, and committed to lifelong learning. On your path to becoming a qualified paramedic, the following are some ideas that will help you achieve success:

Establishing a Study program It is important to establish a study program that allows you sufficient time to review the information included in this book, practice with actual exam questions, and hone your skills. The key to success is consistency.

Utilize a Wide Range of Resources Although this book is an invaluable resource, it is imperative that you augment your study with additional texts, online resources, and practical experience.

Test Your information With the Provided Practice Questions Put your information to the test and hone your analytical thinking skills with the help of the practice questions that are included in this book.

Do Not Hesitate to Seek help: If you find that particular things are difficult to understand or understand, do not be afraid to seek help from more experienced paramedics or professors. They are capable of providing helpful insights and support.

When you are getting close to the end of your preparation, you should try to recreate test settings as precisely as you can by taking practice exams in a setting that is similar to the actual exam. You will gain a better understanding of the structure of the test as well as the limits placed on your time by doing this.

Prepare for the paramedic certification exam carefully, but don't forget to take care of yourself. Make sure you're taking care of both your emotional and physical health at the same time. A healthy lifestyle, getting enough sleep, and learning how to manage stress effectively are all vital.

Learning should be embraced throughout one's life because the path to becoming a paramedic does not end with certification. Make a commitment to learning for the rest of your life and to keeping up with the latest developments in EMS.

The Anatomy and Physiology of the Human Body, Chapter 2

Understanding the complexities of human anatomy and physiology is absolutely necessary for those who work in the field of emergency medical care. When people call for help after suffering serious injuries or experiencing a medical emergency, you, as a paramedic, are often the first person they speak to. You need to have a firm understanding of the structure and function of the human body in order to deliver the highest possible level of care. This chapter digs into the fascinating world of anatomy and physiology, laying the groundwork for you to become an informed and capable paramedic in the process.

The Significance of Anatomy and Physiology in Today's World

Both anatomy and physiology are essential components of the medical field. Anatomy is concerned with the structure of the body, whereas physiology investigates the activities of the body. These two branches of study are linked and complement one another. When taken together, they offer a full picture of the human body and the processes that take place within it. These are the reasons why these topics are so important for paramedics:

Accurate Evaluation: In order to evaluate patients accurately, paramedics must have a strong understanding of anatomy. Knowing the location of organs, muscles, and other structures, as well as the functions they perform, is helpful for paramedics in identifying potential problems and injuries.

Diagnostic Skills In the course of their work, paramedics are frequently tasked with determining the possible diagnoses of patients based on the symptoms and outward manifestations of those diagnoses. Accurate diagnoses and decisions on therapy can be made with the help of an understanding of anatomy and physiology.

Effective Communication The understanding of anatomy and physiology that a paramedic possesses helps them transmit essential information to other medical professionals regarding the status of their patients while they are speaking with them. This guarantees that all of the individuals involved in the care of a patient have the same understanding of the situation.

Clinical Decision-Making: Paramedics are responsible for making crucial decisions while on the job, such as deciding which airway management strategies are the most effective and which drugs to give to patients. These decisions are informed by a deep comprehension of anatomical and physiological principles.

In order to ease a patient's dread and anxiety, it is helpful to explain the patient's illness and therapy in words that are easy to understand. Patients are more likely to place their trust in paramedics who are able to properly communicate medical facts with them.

Recognizing the potential influence that an injury or medical condition may have on other body systems is helpful for paramedics in anticipating and preventing problems.

A Brief Outline of Human Anatomy

The study of the structures that make up the human body, from the tiniest cells to the largest organs, is referred to as human anatomy. It is vital for a paramedic to have an understanding of the anatomical organization of the human body in order to be able to give good care. An outline of the most important aspects of human anatomy is as follows:

Organization on Many Different Levels The human body is organized on many different levels, ranging from the most microscopic to the most macroscopic. Atoms and molecules, cells, tissues, organs, and organ systems are all included in these levels of organization. To truly appreciate anatomy, one must first understand how the different levels interact with one another.

Cavities of the Body The human body is made up of a number of cavities that serve to house and protect the body's critical organs. These are the cranial cavity, which houses the brain, the thoracic cavity, which houses the heart and lungs, and the abdominal cavity, which houses organs such as the stomach, liver, and intestines.

Principal Organ Systems: The human body is made up of a variety of different organ systems, each of which performs a particular job. The cardiovascular system, which includes the heart and blood vessels, the respiratory system, which includes the lungs and airways, the musculoskeletal system, which includes the muscles and bones, and the neurological system, which includes the brain and nerves, are all important systems for paramedics to understand.

Anatomical Planes: In order to accurately describe the body's structures, anatomists use three main planes: the sagittal plane, the frontal (or coronal) plane, and the transverse plane. The sagittal plane divides the body into left and right portions, while the frontal (or coronal) plane divides the body into front and back portions. The transverse plane divides the body into upper and lower sections.

Body Regions: The human body can be broken down into a number of distinct regions to make the study of anatomy more manageable. The head, neck, thorax (chest), abdomen, pelvis, and extremities (arms and legs) are all considered to be a part of these regions.

Definitions of Important Anatomical Terms

In order to precisely explain the structures of the body, anatomy makes use of a highly specialized language. It is absolutely necessary to become familiar with anatomical language in order to communicate and document information effectively in the healthcare field. The following is a list of important anatomical words that you will come across in your work as a paramedic:

The front or forward part of the body is referred to as the anterior (Ventral) region.

Posterior, often known as dorsal, is a term that describes the back or the rear section of the body.

The word "superior" refers to a higher or more prominent position.

The word "inferior" denotes a lower or the lowest possible location.

A structure that is closer to the body's midline is referred to as medial.

A structure that is located laterally relative to the body's midline is said to be lateral.

A structure that is said to be proximal is one that is situated in closer proximity to the place of attachment or origin.

A structure that is further removed from its place of attachment or origin is said to have a distal location.

Superficial refers to structures that are located close to the surface of the body.

Structures that are further beneath the surface of the body are referred to as being "deep."

Structures that are placed in or near the center of an organ or bodily component are indicated by the term "central."

The term "peripheral" is used to describe constructions that are situated on the outside margins or farther away from the center.

Lateral and Medial are terms that are used to denote relative locations to the midline. "Lateral" indicates a position that is farther away from the midline, whilst "Medial" indicates a position that is closer to the midline.

Both superior and inferior are phrases that are used to define the relationship of one structure's location in relation to another structure.

These are phrases that are used to express the relative distance from one structure to another. Proximal and distal are used interchangeably.

The depth of a structure within the body can be described using these terms: superficial, deep, and intermediate.

A Brief Exposition of Human Physiology

The study of how the structures of the body function and how they work together to keep a living organism alive is called physiology. It investigates how the body's many systems are able to keep homeostasis, or the ability to keep an internal environment consistent despite changes in the external environment. When working as a paramedic, it is essential to have a fundamental knowledge of physiology in order to comprehend how the human body reacts to traumatic injuries, sickness, and medical interventions.

The following is a list of important topics of physiology that a paramedic ought to be knowledgeable with:

Homeostasis is the natural process that the body uses to keep its internal environment constant, and it is referred to as homeostasis. It entails managing parameters including the temperature of the body, the pressure in the blood vessels, and the pH levels within specific ranges.

Cellular physiology studies the fundamental building block of life, the cell. Cells are responsible for critical functions such as the creation of energy, the maintenance of ion balance, and the synthesis of proteins.

The nervous system is the part of the body that is in charge of sending messages to and from different parts of the body. It is comprised of the brain and spinal cord, which make up the central nervous system, as well as the nerves that are located outside of the central nervous system, which make up the peripheral nervous system.

The endocrine system is responsible for controlling the functioning of the body by producing hormones and secreting them into the bloodstream. The pituitary, thyroid, and adrenal glands are important components of the endocrine system.

Muscles allow for movement and are responsible for processes such as contracting the heart and passing food through the digestive system. The muscular system includes the skeletal, cardiac, and smooth muscle groups.

The respiratory system is responsible for facilitating gas exchange, which involves the delivery of oxygen to the cells of the body and the removal of carbon dioxide from those cells. It consists of the lungs as well as the airways.

Heart and blood vessels make up what's known as the cardiovascular system, which is made up of the cardiovascular system. It eliminates waste products from the tissues of the body while also delivering oxygen and nutrients to them.

This system is in charge of breaking down and absorbing the nutrients that are contained in food. It is called the gastrointestinal system. It is composed of organs such as the stomach, the small intestine, and the liver.

The renal system, also known as the urinary system, is responsible for filtering the blood, eliminating waste from the body, and maintaining a healthy fluid and electrolyte balance. The kidneys and the bladder are essential organs.

The skin, which is the body's biggest organ, acts as a protective barrier against the environment and is part of the integumentary system. It contributes to the regulation of temperature as well as the sense of heat.

The Body's Blood and Circulatory System

The cardiovascular system is one of the most important aspects of human physiology. The fundamental purpose of this system, which includes the heart, blood vessels, and blood itself, is to carry oxygen, nutrition, hormones, and waste products throughout the body. It is comprised of the cardiovascular system. It is necessary for paramedics to have a solid understanding of the physiology of the circulatory system since they routinely treat patients who are experiencing circulation problems.

The following is a list of the most important parts of the circulatory system:

The heart is a muscular organ that is responsible for pumping blood throughout the body. It is located in the chest. It is made up of four chambers, specifically the left and right atriums, as well as the left and right ventricles.

Arteries, veins, and capillaries are the three subtypes of blood vessels that make up the human circulatory system. At the cellular level, capillaries are responsible for facilitating the exchange of oxygen, nutrients, and waste products. Arteries are responsible for transporting oxygenated blood away from the heart, while veins are responsible for transporting deoxygenated blood back to the heart.

Blood is a crucial fluid that transports oxygen, nutrition, hormones, and waste products throughout the body. Blood is a red color. In addition to this, it plays an important part in the body's immunological response as well as the regulation of temperature. Platelets, red blood cells, and white blood cells are the components that make up blood. Plasma is the liquid component of blood.

Pathways of the Circulatory System The circulatory system has two primary pathways, known respectively as pulmonary circulation and systemic circulation. The lungs are responsible for oxygenating the blood that is carried by pulmonary circulation, whereas oxygenated blood is carried by systemic circulation to all of the body's tissues.

The Processes Involved in Breathing

Another essential component of human physiology is the respiratory system. It performs the necessary job of supplying oxygen to the body as well as eliminating carbon dioxide, which is a byproduct of metabolism. Because respiratory problems are so common in emergency situations, it is especially important for paramedics to have a solid understanding of respiratory physiology.

The following is a list of the most important parts of the respiratory system:

The Lungs: The lungs are the organs that are in charge of breathing and exchanging gases. They are made up of millions of minuscule air sacs known as alveoli, which are the sites where oxygen is absorbed into the bloodstream and carbon dioxide is expelled.

The Airways: The trachea, often known as the windpipe, the bronchi, which are tubes that lead to the lungs, and the bronchioles, which are smaller airways found within the lungs, make up the airways. These structures contribute to the process of air entering and leaving the lungs.

The muscles in the intercostal space and the diaphragm work together to produce the contraction that is necessary for breathing. By contracting, the diaphragm causes the chest cavity to expand, which in turn draws in more air. The exhalation of air occurs when the diaphragm is allowed to relax.

Exchange of Gases: The process of exchanging gases takes place in the alveoli. During this process, oxygen from the air that is inhaled is absorbed into the bloodstream, and carbon dioxide is released from the bloodstream and into the air that is exhaled.

Control of Respiration The respiratory center in the brain is responsible for regulating the rate of breathing as well as the depth of breathing based on parameters such as the levels of oxygen and carbon dioxide in the blood.

The Relationship Between Common Medical Conditions and the Human Body's Anatomy and Physiology

In order to be an effective caregiver as a paramedic, it is essential to have a solid understanding of the ways in which common medical diseases are connected to the anatomical and physiological systems of the human body. The following are some examples:

Infarction of the Myocardium: Also known as a Heart Attack, a Myocardial Infarction happens when the blood supply to the heart muscle is cut off. It is frequently brought on by a narrowing of the coronary arteries, which restricts the flow of blood. It is absolutely necessary to have an understanding of the circulatory system in order to recognize the symptoms and respond effectively.

A stroke, also known as a cerebrovascular accident, occurs when there is an interruption in the normal flow of blood to the brain. This disruption can lead to the death of brain cells. When evaluating and treating stroke patients, knowledge of both the circulatory system and the neurological system is absolutely necessary.

Breathing Difficulties Can Be Caused By Conditions That impact The Respiratory System Conditions that impact the respiratory system, such as asthma, pneumonia, or chronic obstructive pulmonary disease (COPD), can cause breathing difficulties. Assessing and treating these disorders, which include the architecture and physiology of the respiratory system, requires a certain level of expertise on the part of paramedics.

Dehydration: Dehydration can cause electrolyte and fluid imbalances in the body. Dehydration can also lead to fatigue. When diagnosing and treating dehydrated patients, having a solid understanding of the functions of the renal and circulatory systems is absolutely necessary.

Diabetes is a condition in which the body has difficulties controlling the amount of glucose (blood sugar) that is produced. It has a connection to the endocrine system as well as the pancreas, which is responsible for the production of insulin. The symptoms of hypoglycemia and hyperglycemia need to be recognized by paramedics so that they can administer the correct treatment.

Putting It Into Practice: Evaluating Patients

You will frequently be the first person to evaluate patients in severe situations if you are working as a paramedic. The evaluation of a patient is a methodical process that places a significant premium on your understanding of anatomy and physiology. The following is an overview of the process of assessing the patient:

Measure the Scene: Before doing anything else, you should make sure that you are safe and examine the area. Take into account any potential risks, as well as the number of patients involved.

main Survey: The main survey focuses on identifying and treating illnesses that pose an immediate risk to the patient's life. The acronym "ABCs" is frequently employed, with "A" standing for "airway," "B" standing for "breathing," and "C" standing for "circulation." In this stage, you will need to have a comprehensive knowledge of the respiratory and circulatory systems.

Secondary Survey: After all potentially fatal problems have been resolved, it is time to go on to the secondary survey. This requires a thorough evaluation from head to toe, which draws on your knowledge of the anatomy of the human body.

Monitoring of Vital Signs: Be sure to keep an eye on your temperature, as well as your heart rate, blood pressure, and respiration rate. For proper interpretation of vital signs, a fundamental understanding of the circulatory system is required.

Collecting Relevant Medical History: When taking a history, make sure to include any previous diseases, drugs, allergic reactions, and events that led up to the current situation.

Examination of the Patient Carry out a comprehensive evaluation of the patient's physical state, including an assessment of the patient's general appearance, degree of awareness, skin color and condition, and the presence or absence of any apparent injuries. Because you have an understanding of anatomy, you are able to recognize possible problems.

equipment for Diagnosis Collecting extra Information on the Patient Utilize diagnostic equipment like as electrocardiograms (ECGs), pulse oximetry, and blood glucose monitors in order to collect extra information on the patient's state.

contact: Maintaining strong lines of contact with the patient during the entire evaluation process is of the utmost importance. Give an explanation for your actions, get their approval for the treatment, and reassure them.

The Results of the Common Assessment and Their Implications

The ability to recognize and properly interpret assessment findings is an essential skill for paramedics. These findings provide essential information about the patient's condition and aid decision-making regarding therapy. The following is a list of common assessment findings and the ramifications of those findings:

Cyanosis: A bluish coloring of the skin, cyanosis may be an indication of inadequate oxygenation and decreased circulation. It may be an indication that you are having problems with your heart or lungs.

Reduced Consciousness A reduced degree of consciousness may be the result of a number of different events, such as a head injury, a stroke, or low blood sugar. The identification of the problem is absolutely necessary before suitable intervention can be taken.

irregular Heart Rhythms The ability to recognize irregular heart rhythms on an electrocardiogram (ECG) can assist in the diagnosis of cardiac disorders that call for specialized treatment or interventions.

Distress in the Respiratory Tract The presence of signs of respiratory distress, such as rapid or laborious breathing, may be an early warning sign of illnesses such as asthma, pneumonia, or congestive heart failure.

Blood Pressure That Is Too High Hypertension, often known as high blood pressure, can be an early warning sign of more serious health problems, such as cardiovascular disease. It is essential to have an understanding of the circulatory system in order to comprehend the implications of having high blood pressure.

Decreased Oxygen Saturation: A low oxygen saturation level, as measured by pulse oximetry, may signal respiratory or circulatory difficulties that require immediate attention. These conditions can be life-threatening.

The Application of Concepts to Real-World Circumstances

Consider the following examples to better understand the significance of having a strong understanding of anatomy and physiology in the function of a paramedic:

Cardiac Arrest Is the First Possible Outcome

You make your way to the site, where you find a patient who has passed out and is unconscious. When beginning cardiopulmonary resuscitation (CPR) and defibrillation, having a solid understanding of the circulatory system is absolutely necessary. In order to diagnose arrhythmias and evaluate the efficacy of your therapies, you need to have a solid understanding of the anatomy and physiology of the heart.

The second possible outcome is a respiratory emergency.

You have been dispatched to assist a patient who is having significant trouble breathing right now. When evaluating airway patency, breathing patterns, and lung sounds, having knowledge of the anatomy and physiology of the respiratory system is absolutely necessary. Your treatments, such as giving oxygen or providing support for ventilation, will be more effective if you have a solid understanding of the mechanics of breathing.

The third possible outcome is a traumatic injury.

A patient presents at the scene of a car accident with considerable bleeding from a leg wound. The collision was caused by a motor vehicle. Because of your knowledge of the circulatory system, you are able to notice the urgent need to control any bleeding that may be occurring. It is vital to have an understanding of anatomy in order to locate arteries, veins, and other potential causes of bleeding.

Scenario 4: A Critical Diabetes Situation

You have been summoned to aid a patient who appears to be disoriented and bewildered. To be able to recognize the symptoms of hypoglycemia or hyperglycemia, one must have an awareness of the endocrine system and the part that insulin plays in the regulation of blood glucose. Your ability to deliver the appropriate treatment is directly correlated to how well you understand this information.

Enhanced Learning and Development Opportunities

Because paramedicine is a rapidly developing discipline, those who wish to become paramedics are required to demonstrate a dedication to lifelong learning and to keeping abreast of the most recent advances in medical care. Take into consideration, in addition to the education and training you received initially, the following opportunities for professional development:

additional Training: If you want to broaden both your skill set and your career options, you should pursue additional training in a specialty field such as critical care, neonatal care, or pediatric care.

Certification: If you want to improve your qualifications, you need get some more certificates. Some good ones are Advanced Cardiac Life Support (ACLS), Pediatric Advanced Life Support (PALS), and Neonatal Resuscitation Program (NRP).

Conferences and Seminars: It is important to stay current in the field of emergency medicine by attending conferences and seminars in order to learn about the most recent research, treatments, and equipment.

Conducting Research and Publishing Articles Conducting research or publishing articles on EMS-related issues is a great way to contribute to the overall body of knowledge in the field while also advancing your personal understanding.

Mentoring: Programs designed to guide and support new paramedics entering the field should be considered mentorship programs. Giving back to the community in a way that allows you to share your expertise and experience may be quite fulfilling.

The Pharmacology Covered in Chapter 3

The study of pharmacology is an essential part of the practice of paramedicine. In the course of responding to a variety of medical crises, it is your duty as a paramedic to provide patients with a large selection of different medications. For the sake of patient safety, the provision of quality treatment, and the making of educated decisions regarding the administration of medication, having a solid understanding of pharmacology is absolutely necessary. This chapter looks into the field of pharmacology, including topics such as the fundamentals of drug administration, the significance of maintaining a secure medication environment, and the essential pharmaceuticals that are frequently employed in paramedicine.

The Significance of Pharmacology in Today's World

The study of medications and how they interact with the human body is known as pharmacology. The study of how medications are used to prevent, diagnose, and treat medical diseases is included in this field of study. When it comes to delivering prehospital treatment, pharmacology is an extremely important part of the discipline of paramedicine. The following are some of the reasons why paramedics need an understanding of pharmacology:

Medication is frequently an essential part of patient care and is therefore referred to as "patient care." In addition to alleviating pain, managing heart diseases, treating seizure disorders, and treating a range of other medical conditions, they can be used. The ability to understand pharmacology is absolutely necessary in order to provide effective treatment.

In life-threatening situations, it is the responsibility of paramedics to give patients the medications that are necessary to sustain life. When used appropriately, medications like epinephrine, which is delivered to treat severe allergic reactions as well as cardiac arrest, have the potential to save patients' lives.

Pain Management is an important skill for paramedics to have since they frequently encounter patients who are in excruciating pain as a result of their injuries or medical conditions. When it comes to giving efficient pain relief, having knowledge of analgesic medications and how to use them correctly is quite necessary.

Patient Assessment: In order to establish the right drugs and dosages, paramedics are required to perform patient assessments. Because of their knowledge of pharmacology, paramedics are able to make educated choices regarding the medications that are most suited for the specific condition of each individual patient.

Medication Safety: In the field of paramedicine, medication safety is of the utmost importance. In order to reduce the risks connected with the administration of medications, paramedics need to have a thorough understanding of the potential adverse effects, contraindications, and drug interactions.

Communication: It is extremely important to have effective communication with both patients and healthcare providers. It is necessary for paramedics to be able to describe the function of medications, discuss any potential adverse effects, and gain the patient's informed consent before administering any prescription.

Foundational Concepts in Pharmacology

In order to have a firm grip on the fundamentals of pharmacology, it is essential to have a firm grasp on the classification of pharmaceuticals as well as the elements that influence the actions of drugs. The following are some key ideas that are essential to understanding the discipline of pharmacology:

Classifications of Drugs: Drugs are sorted into many categories according to their therapeutic applications and the ways in which they work. Analgesics, often known as pain relievers, bronchodilators, which are used to treat respiratory diseases, and antiarrhythmics, which treat cardiac rhythm issues, are examples of common pharmacological classes.

Medications can be given to a patient in a variety of ways, such as orally (by mouth), intravenously (IV), intramuscularly (IM), subcutaneously (SC), or inhaled. Each of these methods is referred to as a different route of administration. The speed and efficiency with which a medicine takes effect are both impacted by the mode of delivery.

The study of how medications are absorbed by the body, distributed throughout the body, digested, and eliminated from the body is referred to as pharmacokinetics. The study of pharmacokinetics can assist in determining the correct dosage and route of administration for various drugs.

The study of pharmacodynamics focuses on the effects that medications have on the body as well as the mechanisms that are responsible for those effects being produced by the pharmaceuticals. When trying to forecast how a medicine will impact a patient, a solid understanding of pharmacodynamics is absolutely necessary.

The amount of time required for one half of a drug's concentration to be removed from the body is referred to as the drug's "half-life." It is vital to have knowledge of the half-life of a medicine in order to calculate the appropriate dose intervals.

Inappropriateness of a certain medication or treatment for a given patient might be attributed to the presence of certain conditions known as contraindications. In order to prevent giving potentially dangerous drugs to patients, paramedics need to have a solid understanding of contraindications.

Side Effects and Adverse Reactions: Medications have the potential to produce both sides of this coin. Side effects are to be anticipated and may be easily managed, whereas bad reactions are completely unanticipated and could have serious consequences. These side effects need to be identified and managed by the paramedics.

Drug Interactions: Certain medications have the potential to interact with one another and change the effects of both of them. When providing numerous drugs to a patient, paramedics have a responsibility to be aware of and take into account the possibility for adverse drug interactions.

Dosage of Medication It is essential to perform dosage calculations accurately in order to guarantee that patients get the appropriate amount of medication. It is necessary for paramedics to be able to determine dosages depending on a variety of patient characteristics, including age, weight, and condition.

Security of Medication

When it comes to patient care, medication safety is of the utmost importance. In order to ensure that patients receive their prescriptions in a secure manner, paramedics are required to follow a number of specific safety procedures. The following are fundamental guidelines for the safe use of medications:

Check the Orders for Medication: Always perform a second check to guarantee the accuracy of your medicine orders. Verify the drug's name as well as the dosage and the method of administration.

Evaluation of the Patient It is necessary to evaluate the patient in order to determine whether or not the patient should be given medication. Evaluation of vital signs, medical history, allergies, and drugs currently being taken is included in this step.

Administering Medications Correctly: When giving medications, ensure that you do it in accordance with all of the specified protocols and recommendations. Take into consideration the following "rights" when administering medication: the right patient, the right medication, the right dose, the right route, and the appropriate time.

Education of the Patient It is important to educate the patient on the medication that is being given to them, including its function and any possible adverse effects. When it is required, get informed consent from the patient.

Documentation It is crucial to have documentation that is both accurate and comprehensive. Make sure you keep track of the patient's reaction, as well as the medicine, dose, and route that were used. Maintain a record of any unfavorable responses or side effects.

Pharmacological Support: If you have any questions regarding a medicine or how it should be used, you should seek the advice of a medical control physician or a pharmacist.

Labeling of Medications It is imperative that the medication's label be thoroughly examined before it is administered. Check the drug's expiration date to make sure it is consistent with the prescription you have been given.

Medication Administered Intravenously When giving pharmaceuticals intravenously, it is imperative that careful attention be paid to the appropriate dilution and infusion rates. Maintaining proper aseptic technique is essential for avoiding infections.

Always keep a close eye on how the patient is reacting to the drug, and make sure to monitor their response. Prepare yourself to respond appropriately in the event that you experience any unpleasant effects.

Medication Types Commonly Used in Paramedicine

In the field, paramedics come into contact with many different kinds of drugs. Some of these pharmaceuticals are employed in the treatment of particular medical diseases or emergent situations. The following is a list of some of the more common medications that paramedics are trained to administer:

Epinephrine is an essential medicine that is utilized in the treatment of severe allergic responses (anaphylaxis) as well as cardiac arrest. It accomplishes this by narrowing the blood arteries and speeding up the heart rate.

Nitroglycerin is a medication that is prescribed to patients suffering from angina (chest pain) as well as other sorts of cardiac disorders. It does this by relaxing the blood arteries, which in turn improves blood flow to the heart.

Aspirin: Aspirin is used to minimize the risk of blood clot formation and is commonly given to patients who are feeling chest pain or who have a suspicion that they may be having a heart attack.

The bronchodilator known as albuterol is used to treat a variety of respiratory disorders, including asthma and chronic obstructive pulmonary disease (COPD). It does this by relaxing the muscles in the airways, which in turn makes breathing easier.

Glucose: Glucose is used to treat low blood sugar, which is medically referred to as hypoglycemia. Diabetic patients who are experiencing altered mental state or other symptoms are frequently given glucose.

Fentanyl is a highly effective opioid analgesic that is used for the control of pain. In the event of severe pain, such as that caused by fractures or burns, it is given to the patient.

Diazepam is a drug that is prescribed to patients suffering from epileptic seizures and anxiety. It has a calming effect on the nervous system and soothes tense muscles.

Naloxone is a medication that can be administered to a patient in order to reverse the effects of an opioid overdose. It has the ability to quickly restore normal breathing in people who have stopped breathing as a result of the use of opioids.

Amiodarone is a type of antiarrhythmic drug that is prescribed to patients suffering from a variety of irregular heart rhythms. Arrhythmias that pose a significant risk to one's life can be treated with it.

Activated Charcoal: In situations where someone has been poisoned, activated charcoal can be used to inhibit the absorption of hazardous compounds into the bloodstream by absorbing them in the stomach first.

Case Studies: The Effects of Medication on Patients

Consider the following case studies to acquire a deeper comprehension of the various ways in which pharmacology can be applied in the field of paramedicine:

Cardiac Arrest, the First Case Study

You are dispatched to a residence in response to reports that a patient in their middle years has passed out and is unresponsive. After determining that the patient is in cardiac arrest and performing an assessment, you start cardiopulmonary resuscitation, also known as CPR. The administration of epinephrine is a component of advanced life support. Its purpose is to assist in the restoration of circulation and to increase the likelihood of a successful resuscitation. Epinephrine slows blood flow through blood vessels, speeds up the heart rate, and improves coronary perfusion, all of which are essential for individuals who are experiencing cardiac arrest.

Case Study No. 2: Administration of Convulsions

You respond to a 911 call about a patient who is having seizures and arrive at the scene. As soon as you arrive, you notice that the patient is having convulsions while they are having a seizure. After making sure the patient is safe and maintaining their airway, you give them diazepam, which is a drug that helps stop the seizure activity and functions as an anticonvulsant. In order to properly manage the patient's condition, it is essential to have a solid understanding of the pharmacological concepts underlying diazepam.

Case Study Number Three: An Extreme Allergic Reaction

One of our patients was stung by a bee in a nearby park, and as a result, they are having a very difficult time breathing, as well as swelling in their face and hives. You are familiar with the signs of anaphylaxis, a severe allergic reaction that can even be fatal. In this scenario, you would give the patient epinephrine, which has the ability to quickly reverse the allergic response by acting as both a bronchodilator and a vasoconstrictor. Understanding the pharmacology of epinephrine is essential to administering treatment that is both prompt and effective in saving lives.

Case Study No. 4: Ache in the Chest

You go to the location of a patient who has called in complaining of severe chest discomfort. You have a strong suspicion that the patient is experiencing a heart attack (also known as a myocardial infarction) based on their medical history and their symptoms. Aspirin is then given to the patient once the patient's condition has been evaluated and it has been determined that there are no contraindications. The pharmacological effect of aspirin, which involves decreasing platelet aggregation, helps lower the risk of blood clot formation in coronary arteries, which in turn improves the patient's chances of surviving the condition.

Education on Going in the Field of Pharmacology

Because pharmacology is a profession that is constantly undergoing change, paramedics are required to be current on all of the most recent advancements, drugs, and protocols. Continuing education in pharmacology can be accomplished through the following methods:

Participate in continuous training and refresher classes to strengthen your understanding of various medications and how to properly administer them.

Use credible internet resources to gain access to the most recent information about pharmaceuticals and pharmacological breakthroughs. Examples of online resources that fall into this category are educational websites and medical journals.

Pharmacology Updates: Ensure that you are up to date on the latest changes to drug guidelines and practices by following official sources such as your EMS agency or medical control.

Case Reviews: On a consistent basis, evaluate and discuss situations that involve the administration of medication with your coworkers or medical directors in order to gain knowledge from real-world experiences.

Consult with Pharmacists Establishing contacts with pharmacists who can provide helpful insights into the management of medications and answer particular queries is an important step in the process of consulting with pharmacists.

Initiatives Regarding Medication Safety Be a Champion for Medication Safety in Your Organization Be an advocate for medication safety in your organization. Take part in safety programs and make sure to report any events or near misses that are related to medications.

The Pathophysiology of the Condition

Pathophysiology is the study of how diseases and medical conditions arise within the human body and how they affect normal physiological processes. It is also the study of how abnormal physiological processes can lead to disease. When working as a paramedic, having a strong understanding of pathophysiology is essential for identifying, evaluating, and treating a wide variety of different types of medical emergencies. In this chapter, we will discuss the principles of pathophysiology, which is the study of how the body reacts to various illnesses and injuries, and how this information can be applied in your practice as a paramedic.

Pathophysiology's Importance in the Field of Paramedicine

The discipline of pathophysiology acts as a connecting link between normal anatomical structure and the outward manifestations of disease. It comprises the study of both structural and functional changes that occur within the body as a result of various medical disorders, injuries, or environmental variables. These changes can occur as a result of a variety of environmental factors, injuries, or medical conditions. In the context of paramedicine, having a solid understanding of pathophysiology is essential for a number of reasons, including the following:

Recognition and Evaluation: In order to do their jobs effectively, paramedics need to be able to detect the signs and symptoms of a wide variety of injuries and illnesses. You can gain a better understanding of the underlying reasons of various clinical manifestations by having a solid understanding of pathophysiology.

Clinical Decision-Making Paramedics are frequently required to make important and time-sensitive choices while working in the field. Your treatment decisions and treatments should be guided by your knowledge of pathophysiology so that they are appropriate for the patient's condition.

Treatment Efficacy: It is essential, in order to evaluate the effectiveness of treatments and interventions, to have a solid understanding of how the body reacts to them. Understanding the pathophysiology of a condition helps you monitor and modify your interventions appropriately.

Communication: Having a strong foundation in pathophysiology is necessary in order to communicate effectively with both patients and healthcare providers. If you are able to explain a medical issue, its causes, and the reasoning behind your treatment plan to a patient, this can assist create trust and compliance with the treatment plan.

Advocacy for Patients: Paramedics have an essential part to play in the process of advocating for their patients. If you have a strong understanding of pathophysiology, you will have the ability to advocate for care that is both appropriate and timely.

Continuing Education: Because the field of paramedicine is always evolving, it is necessary to continue one's education. The study of pathophysiology is at the heart of many emergency medical services (EMS) educational programs, and it is essential for your continued professional development to remain abreast of any recent advancements in this field.

Concepts Crucial to the Study of Pathophysiology

In order to successfully navigate the complexities of pathophysiology, you need to be conversant with a number of fundamental concepts and principles, including the following:

Etiology is a medical term that describes the root of a disease, often known as the cause. It is possible for it to be infectious (caused by pathogens such as bacteria, viruses, or fungi), genetic (coming from factors inherited), environmental (due to variables such as chemicals or trauma), or idiopathic (of unknown origin).

The process by which a disease first manifests itself and then spreads throughout the body is referred to as its pathogenesis. It is characterized by a chain of occurrences that ultimately results in the clinical indications of the disorder.

Clinical manifestations are the signs and symptoms that can be seen by an observer or are felt by a patient. Clinical manifestations are the result of a disease or condition. These can be objective (measurable, like vital signs), or subjective (reported by the patient, like pain or nausea), depending on the nature of the symptom.

The term "diagnosis" refers to the process of determining the nature of a patient's health problem or disease by analyzing clinical signs, laboratory test results, and imaging investigations. The ability to diagnose a patient paves the way for more focused treatment and management.

A disease's prognosis is an assessment of how the illness is likely to progress in the future. It could be anything from a full recovery to a chronic disease or even a condition that is terminal.

Complications are subsequent conditions or occurrences that can arise as a result of the primary disease. Complications can be referred to as "complications." A severe case of the flu, for instance, can sometimes lead to complications such as pneumonia.

The treatment of a medical illness is determined by its pathophysiology and may involve the use of pharmaceuticals, surgical procedures, adjustments to one's way of life, or other types of interventions.

The Way in Which the Body Reacts to Being Hurt or Sick

In order to recover from illness and damage, the body contains a number of sophisticated and malleable defense mechanisms. To successfully assess and manage patients, it is essential to have a solid understanding of these responses. The following is a list of fundamental ways in which the body reacts to pathology:

Inflammation is a complicated immunological response that can be produced by either tissue damage or an infection. The release of chemical mediators, an increase in blood flow, and the migration of white blood cells to the damaged area are all involved in this process. Redness, heat, swelling, and discomfort are all potential outcomes of inflammation.

Activation of the Immune System The immune system is an essential component of the body's defense mechanism against infectious agents. Immune cells are activated in response to the discovery of a potential danger in order to locate and eliminate the offending agent.

Hormonal Responses: When the body is under stress, whether from illness, injury, or both, hormones are released. The production of the hormone cortisol, for instance, which occurs in response to stress and assists the body in coping with the obstacles, is one example.

Coagulation: When tissues are damaged, it is imperative to have a functioning coagulation system in order to prevent excessive bleeding. Nevertheless, an imbalance in the way this system is regulated might result in thrombosis (the production of clots) and contribute to cardiovascular disease.

Alterations in the Cellular State Ailments of many kinds can bring about cellular alterations. For instance, cancer is characterized by the unchecked proliferation and division of cells, which ultimately results in the formation of tumors.

In response to disturbances in the external world, the body attempts to preserve homeostasis by preserving a constant environment within itself. Homeostasis can be thrown off by pathological circumstances, which can then result in symptoms and problems.

The most common medical conditions and an explanation of their underlying pathophysiology

As a result, paramedics are exposed to a wide variety of medical illnesses, each of which has its own unique pathophysiology. Some instances are as follows:

Myocardial Infarction (also known as a Heart Attack): A heart attack takes place when a coronary artery becomes blocked, which results in a deficiency of oxygen and nutrients being delivered to the heart muscle. This can result in damage to the heart tissue.

A stroke, also known as a cerebrovascular accident, can take place when a blood vessel in the brain either becomes blocked off (which causes an ischemic stroke) or ruptures, which causes a hemorrhagic stroke. The brain's cells are deprived of oxygen and nutrients, leading to cell damage or death.

Asthma: Asthma is a chronic respiratory illness characterized by airway inflammation and tightness. The inflammation results in increased mucus production and bronchoconstriction, making it difficult to breathe.

Diabetes Mellitus: Diabetes is a metabolic illness in which the body has problems controlling blood sugar (glucose) levels. In type 1 diabetes, the immune system attacks the insulin-producing cells in the pancreas, while in type 2 diabetes, the body becomes resistant to insulin.

Acute Renal Failure: Acute renal failure can occur due to various causes, including decreased blood flow to the kidneys, toxins, or severe infection. It leads to impaired kidney function and a buildup of waste products in the blood.

Traumatic Brain Injury: Traumatic brain injuries result from head trauma and can lead to various pathophysiological changes, such as swelling of brain tissue, bleeding, and increased intracranial pressure.

Application to Patient Assessment and Treatment

Paramedics are trained to assess patients systematically, considering both their signs and symptoms and the underlying pathophysiology. This structured approach ensures that patients receive the most appropriate care. Here's how pathophysiology is applied in patient assessment and treatment:

Scene Size-Up: The first step in patient assessment involves assessing the scene for safety and determining the number of patients and their potential conditions based on visible signs.

Primary Survey: The primary survey focuses on assessing and addressing life-threatening conditions. Understanding the pathophysiology of critical conditions like cardiac arrest or severe bleeding guides your immediate interventions.

Secondary Survey: The secondary survey is a comprehensive head-to-toe assessment that explores the patient's clinical manifestations and their potential underlying causes based on pathophysiology.

Vital Signs: Monitoring vital signs such as heart rate, blood pressure, respiratory rate, and temperature is essential. Changes in vital signs can provide clues about the patient's condition and the body's response to illness or injury.

Medical History: Obtaining a medical history helps identify underlying conditions that may contribute to the patient's current presentation. Knowing the pathophysiology of these conditions is crucial for making connections.

Diagnostic Tools: Utilize diagnostic tools such as electrocardiograms (ECGs), pulse oximetry, and blood glucose monitoring to gather additional information about the patient's condition.

Communication: Effective communication with the patient is essential. Explaining your assessment findings, potential diagnoses, and treatment plans is important for obtaining informed consent and establishing rapport.

Case Studies: Applying Pathophysiology in Patient Care

To illustrate the practical application of pathophysiology in patient care, consider the following case studies:

Case Study 1: Stroke

You are dispatched to a residence where a family member has found an elderly patient with slurred speech, facial droop, and weakness on one side of the body. Based on the patient's presentation, you suspect a stroke. Your understanding of stroke pathophysiology informs your assessment and the urgency of transport to a stroke center where time-sensitive interventions may be available.

Case Study 2: Diabetes Complication

You respond to a call for a patient experiencing confusion and shortness of breath. On arrival, you discover that the patient has a history of diabetes and has not been managing their blood sugar levels. The patient's high blood sugar has led to diabetic ketoacidosis (DKA). Your knowledge of the pathophysiology of DKA helps you initiate appropriate treatment, including administering insulin and fluids.

Case Study 3: Trauma

At the scene of a motor vehicle accident, you find a patient with severe head trauma and loss of consciousness. The patient's injuries may involve intracranial bleeding, which you recognize as a potentially life-threatening condition based on your understanding of traumatic brain injury pathophysiology. This knowledge guides your decisions to prioritize rapid transport and maintain the patient's airway.

Continuing Education in Pathophysiology

Paramedics are encouraged to pursue ongoing education and professional development in pathophysiology. Here are some ways to stay updated and deepen your understanding of the subject:

Continuing Education Courses: Attend courses and workshops that focus on pathophysiology, offered by your EMS agency or accredited educational institutions.

Medical Journals and Publications: Read medical journals and research articles that provide the latest insights into disease mechanisms and treatment approaches.

Case Reviews and Discussions: Regularly review and discuss complex cases with colleagues and medical directors to enhance your practical knowledge of pathophysiology.

Online Resources: Explore online resources, including educational websites, medical forums, and interactive learning modules that focus on pathophysiology.

Clinical Rotations: Consider clinical rotations or observation opportunities in healthcare settings to gain hands-on experience in patient care and witness pathophysiology in action.

Advanced Education: Pursue advanced degrees or certifications in fields related to paramedicine or healthcare, such as critical care paramedicine, which delve deeper into pathophysiological concepts.

Evaluation of the Patient, which is Chapter 5

The evaluation of the patient is a fundamental component of paramedicine and serves as the basis for the provision of quality prehospital care. It is essential for you as a paramedic to be able to make educated decisions, provide appropriate treatments, and ultimately improve patient outcomes if you are able to conduct patient assessments in a methodical and precise manner. This chapter goes into the art and science of assessing patients, covering everything from the importance of keeping the scene secure to the steps involved in compiling a detailed medical history.

The Importance of Conducting an Evaluation of the Patient

The process of patient assessment is a multi-step procedure that enables paramedics to obtain essential information about a patient's condition, develop alternative diagnoses, and implement treatment strategies that are suitable for the patient's condition. It is impossible to exaggerate the significance of performing a patient assessment in paramedicine:

Life maintain: When a patient's life is in danger, an assessment of the patient is performed to direct immediate actions to maintain essential functions. These interventions include managing the airway, performing cardiopulmonary resuscitation (CPR), and controlling bleeding.

Help with Diagnosis: The assessment process assists paramedics in determining the source of a patient's symptoms, which paves the way for more precise diagnoses and more effective treatments.

Monitoring: Regular patient evaluation enables paramedics to monitor changes in the patient's state. This allows the paramedics to ensure that interventions continue to be effective and that new problems are discovered as soon as possible.

The evaluation of potential dangers at the site is an essential component of the assessment procedure. This helps to ensure that both the patient and the medical staff remain healthy during the process.

Communication: The findings of a comprehensive evaluation are the foundation for effective communication with patients, their families, and the healthcare personnel who care for them. It helps to create rapport, acquire informed consent, and build confidence in the relationship.

Documentation: The results of a comprehensive evaluation are essential for producing accurate and exhaustive documentation, which bolsters efforts to enhance quality of care and maintain continuity of treatment.

The Elements That Comprise a Patient Evaluation

An in-depth patient assessment is made up of a number of essential parts that, when put together, offer a complete picture of the patient's health status. These components are often arranged into a systematic method, which can differ from region to region but typically contains the parts listed below:

The first step in the appraisal procedure is to conduct a comprehensive investigation of the scene in question. The paramedic will determine the mechanism of damage or the nature of the sickness, as well as detect any potential threats, while also ensuring their own safety as well as the patient's.

Primary Survey: The primary survey is a condensed assessment that is primarily concerned with locating and eliminating imminent dangers to human life. The ABCDE strategy, which stands for airway, breathing, circulation, disability, and exposure, is the one that is commonly followed while doing so. During this stage, the most important interventions are given priority.

Monitoring vital indicators such as heart rate, respiration rate, blood pressure, and temperature is an extremely important part of any medical treatment. Alterations in a patient's vital signs can provide early indications of both the state of the patient and the efficacy of the treatments being administered.

Taking a Patient's History It is absolutely necessary to obtain a thorough patient history in order to have a grasp of the patient's medical history, as well as their present symptoms, prescriptions, allergies, and recent occurrences. The SAMPLE acronym, which stands for Signs and Symptoms, Allergies, Medications, Past Medical History, Last Oral Intake, and Events Leading to the Present Illness (or Injury), may be included in the patient's history.

Focused Physical Examination: A complete physical examination from head to toe will help determine whether or not there are any injuries, anomalies, or medical concerns. The inspection needs to be thorough and methodical, beginning at the head and working its way down to the feet.

Diagnostic Tools In order to acquire further information about the patient's state, make use of diagnostic tools such as electrocardiograms (ECGs), blood glucose monitoring, pulse oximetry, and others.

Clinical Decision-Making The information obtained during the assessment is used by paramedics to create differential diagnoses, develop a treatment plan, and make decisions regarding transfer.

Reassessment It is important to continually reassess the patient in order to check for any changes in their condition. This will help to ensure that therapies continue to be successful and suitable.

Taking Stock of the Situation and Conducting a Risk Analysis

The first steps in the process of evaluating a patient involve sizing up the scene and conducting a safety assessment. These steps are absolutely necessary for safeguarding the patient's well-being as well as the safety of the paramedic team. The following are some of the most important things to think about when doing a scene size-up:

Safety at the site: Make sure that you, your team, and the patient are all safe while you are at the site. Always be aware of your surroundings and keep an eye out for potential threats such as traffic, environmental hazards, and aggressive people.

Determine the cause of the patient's condition or damage, often known as the mechanism of the injury or the nature of the illness. This information helps to discover probable injuries or medical conditions by providing context for your examination and assisting in the determination of whether or not they exist.

Number of Patients: Determine whether there are numerous patients and arrange the care you provide in the appropriate order if there are multiple patients. In situations involving a large number of casualties, triage may be required.

Determine whether extra resources, such as additional ambulances, firefighters, law enforcement, or specialized medical teams, are required by determining whether or not further resources are required.

Personal Protective Equipment (PPE): Make sure that you and everyone else on your team are wearing the right PPE to protect against the possibility of contracting an infectious disease or being exposed to dangerous materials.

Materials That Could Be Hazardous Always be on the lookout for potentially hazardous materials that could put both the patient and the responders in danger. If it's safe to do so, evacuate the area.

Methodology for the Primary Survey: ABCDE

The ABCDE method is utilized in the primary survey, which is carried out as soon as the scope of the scene has been evaluated. This helps to detect and systematically resolve any urgent hazards to life. Taking this strategy will ensure that steps to support life are started as quickly as possible. The following is an explanation of the ABCDE strategy:

Assess whether or not the patient's airway is patent by doing an airway assessment. Make sure that there are no obstructions in the way and that it is clear. If there is a problem with the airway, the right steps need to be taken to open it and keep it open. These steps include moving the patient's head and employing airway adjuncts such as an oropharyngeal or nasopharyngeal airway.

B - Breathing: Conduct a thorough assessment of the patient's breathing to determine whether or not adequate and efficient ventilation is present. This involves looking for a rise and fall in the patient's chest, listening for sounds associated with breathing, and looking for indicators of respiratory difficulties or discomfort.

C - Circulation: Conduct a thorough assessment of the patient's circulatory system to establish the degree to which it is working properly. Examining the pulse, the heart rate, the blood pressure, and the color of the skin are all components of this step. If the circulation is not functioning properly, you should immediately begin life-saving procedures such as cardiopulmonary resuscitation (CPR) or controlling the bleeding.

Evaluating the patient's neurological status, including their level of consciousness, responsiveness, and pupil reactivity, is part of the diagnostic process for the disability category "D." Examine the individual for any indications of a handicap, such as a change in their mental status, focal neurological deficiencies, or indications of a head injury.

E - Exposure/Environment: Make sure the patient is exposed to the appropriate environment so that you may evaluate them for any injuries or medical issues. Consider environmental aspects, such as the possibility of the patient being exposed to severe temperatures, and respond accordingly to ensure the patient's comfort and safety.

The initial survey is intended to be quick and laser-focused, with the goal of locating and eliminating imminent dangers to life within a matter of minutes. During the initial survey, initiatives that could save lives are put into action. After the initial survey has been finished, the paramedics may move on to the secondary survey in order to collect further information regarding the patient's condition.

Evaluation of the Patient's Vital Signs

The patient's vital signs are essential in determining the general health and stability of the patient. They offer extremely helpful information regarding the patient's physiological status as well as their response to disease or injury. The following are the four basic markers of a person's vitality:

Assessing cardiac function involves taking the individual's heart rate and converting it into beats per minute (bpm). The range of 60-100 beats per minute that is considered typical for people is subject to change depending on factors such as age, physical condition, and medical history.

Rate of Respiration: The rate of breathing, measured in breaths per minute, is used to determine whether or not there is sufficient ventilation. When individuals are at rest, their normal respiratory rate ranges anywhere from 12 to 20 breaths per minute.

Blood Pressure: Blood pressure, which is measured in millimeters of mercury (mmHg), is an evaluation of the force that blood exerts on the arterial walls. Blood pressure is measured in the form of systolic/diastolic, such as 120/80 mmHg. Blood pressure is often represented as systolic (the pressure during heartbeats) over diastolic (the pressure between heartbeats), and it is typically expressed as systolic over diastolic.

Temperature: The thermoregulation of the body can be understood better with the help of the body's temperature, which can be measured in degrees Fahrenheit (°F) or degrees Celsius (°C). The average temperature of an adult's body is roughly 98.6 degrees Fahrenheit (37 degrees Celsius).

The Primary Survey and Its Corresponding Vital Signs in Operation

Take a look at the following example to see how the primary survey and vital signs are employed while assessing a patient:

When you arrive at the scene of an automobile accident, you find a patient who has been thrown from their vehicle. The patient is in critical condition. The patient is lying on the floor and is unresponsive to any stimuli.

The primary survey, often known as the ABCDE method:

You perform a brief examination of the patient's airway and discover that it is partially clogged by blood and vomit. You will use suction to clear the airway, and then you will place an oropharyngeal airway in order to keep it open.

B - Breathing: When you check to see if the patient is breathing, you find that they are not doing so on their own accord. You begin rescue breathing by providing positive pressure ventilation using a device that consists of a bag-valve-mask combination.

When you check the patient's pulse, you notice that it is quite weak and thready. You are concerned about the patient's circulation. The patient's blood pressure cannot be felt by the attending physician. You immediately begin chest compressions and ventilations (CPR) and call for further help as well as an automated external defibrillator (AED).

You continue to administer cardiopulmonary resuscitation for the patient while also monitoring their neurological state. The patient is unresponsive and has pupils that are dilated, which indicates a serious loss in neurological function.

You make sure that the patient is exposed to the appropriate environment so that you can check for injuries. E stands for "exposure" and "environment." You also evaluate the surroundings in terms of its possible dangers and levels of safety.

Evaluation of the Patient's Vital Signs:

In order to obtain an electrocardiogram (ECG), you first measure the patient's heart rate by attaching a cardiac monitor to their chest. The presence of asystole, also known as the absence of cardiac activity, is shown on the monitor, which proves that continued resuscitation attempts are required.

Counting the ventilations that have been administered when performing rescue breathing and noting that the patient is not breathing on their own allows you to determine the patient's respiratory rate.

Blood Pressure: A stethoscope and a manual blood pressure cuff are used to obtain a reading of the patient's blood pressure. There is no discernible change in the blood pressure.

Temperature: Given the serious severity of the patient's illness, it is not a priority to measure the patient's body temperature at this point in the process.

The Making of History

An essential part of performing an assessment on a patient is collecting as much information as possible regarding their medical history. The patient's medical history contains critical information regarding the patient's previous medical issues, current symptoms, prescriptions, allergies, and the circumstances that led up to the patient's current sickness or injury. When taking a patient's medical history, it is common practice to use the abbreviation SAMPLE:

Signs and Symptoms: To start, you should inquire with the patient about any current symptoms they may be experiencing. The patient should be encouraged to describe their symptoms and sensations, such as any discomfort, shortness of breath, dizziness, or weakness they may be experiencing.

In the case of allergies, it is important to enquire about any known allergies, particularly those that are tied to specific medications or environmental variables. Having an allergy can have a substantial influence on the therapy options available.

drugs: You should inquire with the patient about the drugs that they are presently taking. Keep a record of the names of the medications, the dosages, and the number of times they were taken.

Investigate the patient's medical history, which should include any chronic ailments, surgical operations, or hospitalizations that the patient may have had in the past. The patient's medical history from the past can shed light on the underlying health problems.

Find out when the patient last consumed anything by mouth, such as food or drink. When the patient had their last mouthful of food or liquid can be relevant to a variety of medical diseases and procedures.

Inquire with the patient or any witnesses about the circumstances that led up to the current illness or injury. Inquire with the patient or any witnesses about the circumstances that led up to the current predicament. When evaluating the patient's health and deciding how best to treat them, it is critical to have a solid understanding of how the sickness or injury developed.

Examination of the Body with Specialized Attention

A focused physical examination is an in-depth investigation of the patient's body that is conducted with the intention of locating any injuries, anomalies, or illnesses that may be present. The examination is often performed in a head-to-toe manner, in which each body part is evaluated one after the other in sequential order. The following are important aspects that should be looked out for during the focused physical examination:

Head and Neck: Conduct a thorough examination of the head and neck, looking for any evidence of injury, deformity, or trauma. Examine the patient's eyes, ears, nose, and mouth, as well as their range of motion in the neck, and look for signs of facial trauma.

Check the chest and abdomen for any injuries, pain, or tenderness. Pay particular attention to the chest. Pay attention to the sounds of the patient's breath and keep an eye out for any indicators of respiratory distress.

Back and Spine: Perform a thorough examination of the back and spine, looking for any injuries or abnormalities. Examine the patient for any evidence of pain, soreness, or spinal cord injury.

Upper Extremities: Visually inspect and physically check for any injuries, abnormalities, or fractures in the patient's arms and hands. Investigate whether or if the fingers have mobility, feeling, and circulation.

Lower Extremities: Conduct a thorough examination of the patient's legs and feet, looking for any fractures, abnormalities, or injuries. Examine the circulation as well as the movement and sensation in the toes.

Examine the patient's pelvis for any signs of injury, instability, or pain. Take into consideration the possibility of pelvic fractures.

Genitourinary and Rectal: Genitourinary and rectal examinations should only be performed when suggested by the patient's state, history, or mechanism of damage. These examinations include looking in the patient's genital and rectal areas.

The targeted physical examination is suited to the patient's situation, and it should be comprehensive while still being time-efficient. During the examination, paramedics have a duty to pay close attention for any indicators of distress, pain, or a change in the patient's mental status.

Instruments for Diagnosis

In order to get new knowledge on a patient's condition, paramedics make use of a wide variety of diagnostic equipment. The evaluation process is aided by these instruments, and certain medical disorders can more accurately be diagnosed as a result. The following are examples of diagnostic instruments that are frequently utilized in prehospital care:

An electrocardiogram, often known as an ECG, is a test that records and monitors the electrical activity of the heart. This aids in the diagnosis of arrhythmias, as well as ischemia and cardiac events.

Pulse oximetry: a pulse oximeter is a device that monitors the oxygen saturation of a patient's blood. This provides information about the amount of oxygen that is being delivered to the patient's tissues.

Monitoring Blood Glucose Blood glucose monitoring is the process of determining the levels of sugar in a patient's blood and is especially crucial for individuals who have diabetes or whose mental status has been disturbed.

Capnography is a method that measures the levels of end-tidal carbon dioxide (EtCO2) in an individual's exhaled breath. It is useful for determining the level of ventilation and verifying the positioning of the endotracheal tube.

Monitoring Blood Pressure Cuffs that either manually or automatically measure blood pressure are referred to as blood pressure monitors. Maintaining a consistent monitoring schedule is essential for tracking changes in the circulatory condition.

The Glasgow Coma Scale, abbreviated as "GCS," is a tool for evaluating a patient's degree of consciousness and neurological function. The GCS is a neurological assessment instrument.

Making Clinical Decisions and Decisions Regarding Transportation

Clinical decisions, differential diagnoses, and treatment plans are developed with the help of the information that is acquired during the patient assessment that is performed by paramedics. The process of making decisions in a clinical setting is an ongoing one that includes the following essential steps:

The process of developing a differential diagnosis involves the paramedics compiling a list of potential diagnoses for the patient based on the patient's signs and symptoms. This list, which is referred to as the differential diagnosis, helps guide decisions on treatment.

Treatment Priorities: Treatments are prioritized based on the state of the patient and the seriousness of their injuries or illnesses. Priority is given to treating diseases that pose a risk to life.

The implementation of therapy entails the beginning of any and all treatments and interventions that are deemed necessary by the state of the patient. This may include the administration of drugs, the provision of oxygen, the immobilization of fractures, or the performance of surgical procedures involving the airway.

Decisions Regarding Transport Paramedics evaluate whether or not patient transport is necessary and decide where to take the patient. The clinical status of the patient, the proximity of specialist care facilities, and an estimate of the amount of time it will take to transport the patient all play a role in the decision-making process.

Evaluation once more

The process of reevaluating a patient is an ongoing one that entails monitoring the patient's condition in a methodical and consistent manner at predetermined time intervals. Reevaluation ensures that therapies continue to be effective while also ensuring that any newly emerging problems are quickly recognized and treated. The following are important components of the reassessment of patients:

Monitoring of Vital Signs: At predetermined time intervals, vital signs should be monitored, including the patient's heart rate, respiration rate, blood pressure, and oxygen saturation levels.

Clinical state: You should continually evaluate the patient's clinical state, which should include their degree of consciousness, their level of pain, and any signs that they are in distress.

Evaluating the effectiveness of treatments and interventions is part of the treatment efficacy process. When necessary, make any necessary adjustments or alterations.

Documentation: Be sure to document the findings of any reassessments, any changes in the patient's condition, as well as any new therapies or interventions.

Maintain open lines of communication with the patient as well as other members of the patient's healthcare team, alerting them of any shifts in the patient's condition or treatment strategy.

Decisions Regarding Transportation: Take into account the results of the patient's reassessment when making transportation decisions. In the event that the patient's condition deteriorates, they may need to be transferred to a different facility or have access to more resources.

Case Studies: Examples of Patient Evaluation in Action

Consider the following case studies as illustrations of how the practical use of patient evaluation might be put into practice:

Case Study No. 1: A Heart-Related Crisis

You go to the location of a patient who is complaining of chest pain and assess the situation. As soon as you get there, you assess the situation, make sure everyone is safe, and then you approach the patient. The patient is aware of their surroundings and cognizant, but they are complaining of acute chest discomfort that has been going on for the previous half an hour. You perform an initial survey on the patient and find that their airway is clear, that they are breathing adequately, and that there are no immediate indicators that their circulation is being compromised. You take a patient's vital signs and find that their heart rate is 110 beats per minute, their respiratory rate is 20 breaths per minute, their blood pressure is 150 over 90, and their oxygen saturation is 98%. The patient's skin has a whitish appearance and is sweating heavily (diaphoretic). You construct a differential diagnosis of acute coronary syndrome (ACS) based on the patient's history and the findings of your assessment, and you immediately begin therapy with oxygen and aspirin. You decide to get an electrocardiogram to verify the diagnosis.

Study No. 2: A Severe Accidental Injury

You are dispatched to a motor vehicle collision where there has been a reported ejection. Upon arrival, you assess the situation to determine how safe it is for your team and do a scene size-up. The patient is lying on the floor and is unresponsive to any stimuli. During the main survey, you notice that the patient has a blocked airway. As a result of the patient's weak pulses and lack of blood pressure, you begin performing cardiopulmonary resuscitation (CPR). The following are the patient's vital signs: heart rate of 40 beats per minute, respiration rate of 0 breaths per minute, blood pressure that is undetectable, and oxygen saturation of 82%. You carry on with CPR and ask for advanced life support (ALS) as well as an automated external defibrillator (AED). You have reason to believe that the patient experienced traumatic cardiac arrest based on the mechanism of injury as well as their presentation, so you begin resuscitation.

Education on Going in Patient Evaluations (Continuing)

The subject of patient evaluation is one that is constantly undergoing change; as a result, paramedics are strongly urged to participate in ongoing education and professional development in order to be up to date on the most effective methods. Your ability to assess patients can be improved in a number of ways, including the following:

Participate in Continuing Education Programs by Attending Workshops and Courses Offered by Your Local Emergency Medical Services Agency or Other Accredited Educational Institutions. Most of the time, these classes will concentrate on more advanced evaluation methods and new developments in patient care.

Training with Simulation: Participate in high-fidelity simulation activities that simulate situations that could occur in real life. The opportunity to put one's knowledge of patient evaluation to the test in a safe and supervised setting is provided through simulation training.

Reassessment on a frequent Basis: It is important to review and update your understanding of patient assessment abilities on a frequent basis by participating in skill drills. One can accomplish this task on their own or in a group environment with other professionals.

Clinical Rotations: Take into consideration the possibility of completing clinical rotations or seeing patients in a variety of medical settings, such as emergency rooms or intensive care units, in order to broaden your experience with a variety of patient situations and evaluation strategies.

Review by Peers and Case Studies: In this activity, you will work with your coworkers to discuss difficult instances and offer your views. Case studies and group discussions with the opinions of peers both present excellent educational opportunities.

Education at a Higher Level: If you want in-depth understanding of patient evaluation procedures and principles, you should pursue education at a higher level, such as advanced degrees or certificates in subjects linked to paramedicine or healthcare.

The Airway and the Breathing Process, Chapter 6

The maintenance of an open airway and normal breathing are essential aspects of patient care in paramedicine. It is essential for the health of patients to have the ability to create and keep open a patent airway, to guarantee adequate oxygenation and ventilation, and to identify and treat respiratory distress or failure. In this chapter, we will discuss the architecture of the respiratory system, the evaluation of the airway and breathing, as well as the techniques and treatments that paramedics use to address difficulties with the airway and breathing.

The Value of Maintaining Proper Airway and Respiratory Function

Both the airway and the act of breathing are vitally important physiological processes because they enable the body to take in oxygen (O2) for the process of metabolism and expel carbon dioxide (CO2), which is a waste product of metabolism. These mechanisms are essential for preserving the body's acid-base balance and delivering oxygen to its tissues and organs in order to ensure proper functioning.

In the field of paramedicine, the significance of the airway and breathing becomes clear in a number of different ways:

Establishing and maintaining a patent airway while also providing appropriate ventilation is one of the most important aspects of life support in the event that a patient is in a potentially fatal circumstance.

Protecting the Airway Doing so helps reduce the risk of aspirating secretions, blood, or vomit into the lungs, which could result in serious respiratory distress or infection.

Distress and Failure of the Respiratory System Recognizing and treating patients who are experiencing respiratory distress or failure as a result of trauma or medical disorders is one of the key responsibilities of paramedics.

Evaluation: The evaluation of the patient's airway and breathing is an important part of the evaluation process. This part of the evaluation helps paramedics identify and address abnormalities that may require rapid interventions.

The Structure and Function of the Respiratory System

It is necessary to have an understanding of the anatomy of the respiratory system in order to comprehend the airways and the act of breathing. The respiratory system is made up of a number of different structures, all of which cooperate with one another to make the exchange of oxygen and carbon dioxide possible. The following are the essential components:

Inhaled air travels through the nasal cavity, which serves as a route for this air. Before it enters the lungs, the air is processed through a filter, it is humidified, and it is warmed.

The pharynx is the part of the upper respiratory tract that connects the nasal cavity to the trachea. It acts as a passageway for both the air and the food that passes through it.

The larynx, often known as the voice box, is situated at the base of the throat, just below the pharynx. It is essential to the process of phonation, which is the act of making sound, and contains the vocal cords.

The trachea is a tube that connects the larynx to the bronchi. This tube is called the trachea. It is protected by cartilaginous rings and lined with ciliated mucous membranes, both of which assist in clearing debris from the airway and keep it open.

Bronchi: The trachea divides into two bronchi, which in turn lead to the right lung and the left lung, respectively. Each bronchus will eventually branch off into several bronchioles as it continues to develop.

Lungs: The lungs are the principal organs that are involved in the process of breathing. They are made up of millions of minuscule air sacs known as alveoli, which are the sites where gas exchange takes place.

The diaphragm is a sheet of muscle that lies between the chest cavity and the abdominal cavity. It acts as a barrier between the two cavities. In the process of breathing, it contracts so that the thoracic cavity can be expanded during inhalation. This is an important function of the diaphragm.

Evaluation of the Airway

The evaluation of the patient's airway is an essential part of the overall evaluation process. Examining the patency (openness) of the airway and looking for any injuries or obstructions are also necessary steps in the process. The following are the primary stages of the airway assessment process:

Before approaching the patient to evaluate their airway, you should first make sure the scene is safe and then approach the patient. Determine the potential risks and take measures to reduce them.

Positioning: Place the patient in a position that will allow for the greatest possible expansion of their airway. It may be necessary to do manual movements to open the airway or to position the patient so that they are lying on their back.

Look, Listen, and Feel: When evaluating the patient's airway, it is important to first observe the patient's breathing, then listen for sounds of breathing, and then feel for air movement. Keep an eye out for indications that the individual is having trouble breathing, such as the use of auxiliary muscles, stridor (a high-pitched sound that can be heard during inhalation), or nasal flaring.

Find and remove any obstructions that may be present in the airway. Obstructions. The tongue, vomit, blood, or foreign objects are some of the most common causes of blockages. To open the airway, you can try procedures such as tilting the head back, lifting the chin, or pushing the jaw forward.

Examine for symptoms of Trauma: When examining the patient for symptoms of trauma to the airway, look for things like blood, edema, or abnormalities. If there is a risk of neck injury, it is imperative that appropriate precautions be taken to protect the cervical spine.

Interventions in the Airway

During the examination, if an airway obstruction or trouble breathing is discovered, the paramedics must immediately implement actions that are appropriate for the situation in order to guarantee proper ventilation and oxygenation. The following are examples of common airway interventions:

Maneuvers for the Airway:

Head-Tilt, Chin-Lift: To perform this procedure, tilt the patient's head backward while simultaneously lifting their chin up. It assists in correcting the alignment of the airway and makes breathing easier.

Jaw Thrust: The jaw thrust maneuver is utilized in situations in which there is a potential for an injury to the cervical spine. It entails raising the patient's jaw while keeping the patient's head and neck in their normal positions.

Airways of the Oral and Nasopharyngeal Cavities:

Oropharyngeal Airway (OPA): An OPA is a curved device that is put into the mouth of the patient in order to prevent the patient's tongue from obstructing the airway.

Nasopharyngeal Airway (NPA): A Nasopharyngeal Airway (NPA) is a device that is put through the nostril to create a clear path for air. When the patient is unable to tolerate an OPA, it is frequently utilized as an alternative.

Suctioning is a procedure that is used to clear the airway of any mucus, blood, or vomit that may be present. Suction devices are utilized by paramedics in order to properly clear the airway.

Devices for the Supraglottic Airway Supraglottic airway devices, such as the King LT or the laryngeal mask airway (LMA), are utilized in situations where conventional airway techniques and adjuncts are unable to provide the desired results. These devices form a seal in the upper airway, which makes it possible to ventilate using positive pressure.

Intubation Through the Trachea The procedure known as endotracheal intubation includes placing a tube into the trachea in order to maintain the patient's airway. It is carried out by paramedics who have completed further training.

Surgical Airway: In the most severe instances of airway obstruction or failure, a surgical airway procedure, such as a cricothyrotomy or tracheostomy, may be carried out to create a direct access to the airway.

Evaluation of the Breathing

Assessing breathing entails determining the nature and magnitude of ventilation's contribution to the process. The following are important components of the breathing assessment:

Counting the number of breaths that you take in one minute will give you an estimate of your respiratory rate. The average adult takes between 12 to 20 breaths per minute, which is considered to be a normal respiratory rate.

Assess the depth of each breath, making a mental note of whether or not it is a shallow or a deep one. It's possible that shallow breathing is a sign of respiratory distress.

Pattern: Pay attention to the patient's breathing pattern and check to see if it is regular, irregular, or if it exhibits any aberrant patterns such as agonal respirations (gasping).

Consider the amount of work that is required to maintain normal breathing. The usage of accessory muscles or retractions (a visible pulling in of the chest or neck) are two signs that may be present if the amount of work that is done during breathing has increased.

During auscultation, a stethoscope is used to listen to the patient's breath sounds. Abnormal breath sounds could be an indication of a problem with the lungs or the airways.

Use of Accessory Muscles It is important to determine whether or not the patient is making use of accessory muscles, such as those in the neck or the sternocleidomastoid, in order to assist with breathing.

Check for symmetry in the movement of your chest during inhalation and exhalation to ensure proper breathing technique. Asymmetry could be a sign of an injury or a problem with the neuromuscular system.

Interventions Regarding Breathing

During the examination, paramedics are required to begin measures in order to treat any irregularities or issues with breathing that are discovered. These interventions must also support sufficient oxygenation and ventilation. The following are examples of common breathing interventions:

Oxygen Administration: Provide the patient with supplemental oxygen in order to raise the amount of oxygen that is present in their blood. Several other delivery systems, such as nasal cannulas, non-rebreather masks, and positive-pressure breathing, are all viable options for oxygen supply.

Ventilation: Positive-pressure ventilation entails aiding the patient's breathing by providing breaths through the use of a bag-valve-mask (BVM) system. This type of ventilation is performed by a healthcare professional. When the patient is unable to breathe effectively on their own, this technique is utilized.

Chest Seal: Patients who have open chest wounds or pneumothorax (collapsed lung) benefit from having a chest seal applied to the wound as it prevents air from entering the pleural space. This is accomplished by placing the chest seal to the wound.

medicine It may be necessary to administer medicine, such as bronchodilators or analgesics, in order to alleviate the patient's pain and minimize the amount of effort required for breathing.

Endotracheal intubation is a type of intubation that includes inserting an endotracheal tube into the trachea in order to stabilize the patient's airway and enable regulated ventilation.

Chest decompression involves inserting a needle or a catheter into the chest of a patient suffering from tension pneumothorax in order to free any trapped air and return the patient's lungs to their normal functioning state.

Stress on the Respiratory System and Inability to Breathe

A core competency for paramedics is the ability to identify respiratory distress and failure and to manage these conditions. The symptoms of respiratory distress include an increase in the amount of effort required to breathe as well as trouble moving air in and out of the lungs. The following are examples of signs and symptoms commonly associated with respiratory distress:

Rapid breathing is referred to as tachypnea.

Utilization of the body's auxiliary muscles

The nostrils become more prominent.

Cyanosis, also known as having blue-colored skin or mucous membranes

Anxiety or a state of agitation

Failure of the respiratory system to sustain enough levels of oxygenation and ventilation can lead to the condition known as respiratory failure. It can be divided into two distinct categories, namely:

Hypoxemic respiratory failure is a form of respiratory failure that is distinguished by low oxygen levels in the blood (hypoxemia) despite having normal or low levels of carbon dioxide in the blood. Pneumonia, pulmonary edema, or severe asthma are some of the factors that might lead to this syndrome.

Hypercapnic Respiratory Failure Hypercapnic respiratory failure, also known as hypercapnia, is characterized by increased levels of carbon dioxide in the blood and is most commonly caused by conditions that restrict airflow, such as chronic obstructive pulmonary disease (COPD) or neuromuscular abnormalities.

When treating respiratory distress or failure, it is important to first identify and treat the underlying cause of the condition, then work to improve oxygenation and ventilation, and finally, provide breathing support as required.

Case Studies: Obstacles in the Airway and the Respiratory System

Consider the following case examples to explain how the theoretical concepts of airway and breathing assessment and therapies might be used in real life:

Case Study No. 1: Obstruction of the Airway

You are dispatched to the scene of an adult patient who is choking. You discover the patient sitting upright, with their hand around their throat, and they are unable to communicate when you arrive. You are aware of the symptoms that indicate a partial obstruction of the airway. You give the patient instructions to keep coughing because you believe this will assist in removing the foreign object that is blocking their airway. The patient's condition continues to deteriorate, and they are unable to cough as a result. You conduct abdominal thrusts, also known as the Heimlich technique, to clear the obstruction. This results in the expulsion of a foreign item, which enables the patient to breathe normally again. You will continue to observe the patient in order to look for any indications of respiratory distress or problems.

Case Study No. 2: An Acute Exacerbation of Asthma

You are on your way to a patient's home when the dispatcher tells you that the patient is having an asthma flare-up. You encounter a woman who is 45 years old and is clearly in a state of distress when you get at the scene. She is wheezing audibly and is using her auxiliary muscles to help her breathe. Her breathing is laborious. Her oxygen saturation is 88 percent while she is breathing in room air, and her respiratory rate is 28 breaths per minute. You provide the patient with reassurance while also beginning treatment with bronchodilators and administering supplemental oxygen. You keep an eye on her breathing as well as her oxygen saturation, and you record how she is responding to the treatment.

Case Study No. 3: Traumatic Pneumothorax Caused by Tension

A patient who was engaged in a high-speed collision is the one you find when you get at the site of an auto accident. The patient is aware of their surroundings but is having significant difficulty breathing. During your examination of the patient's breathing, you notice a reduction in the sounds of breathing on one side of the chest, as well as a deviation of the trachea away from the wounded side. You have a suspicion that the patient has a tension pneumothorax, which is a potentially fatal condition in which air collects in the pleural space and presses on the lung. You swiftly introduce a needle into the chest in order to relieve the tension, and then you let out the air that was trapped there. After noticing an improvement in the patient's respiration, you make arrangements for the patient to be sent to a trauma center for additional evaluation and treatment.

Education on Going in the Field of Airways and Breathing

There is a strong emphasis placed on ongoing education and professional development for paramedics, particularly in the areas of airway and breathing care. Maintaining current knowledge of the most recent recommendations and best practices is absolutely necessary in order to provide high-quality care to patients. You can improve your skills in breathing and airway passages by doing the following:

Training in Advanced Airway Management It is important to consider training in advanced airway management, which may include endotracheal intubation and the implantation of a supraglottic airway device. Additional credentials could be necessary to demonstrate competency in these areas.

Courses Relating to Critical Care Paramedicine: Investigate the possibility of enrolling in critical care paramedicine-related courses, which offer a more in-depth look into advanced airway management and mechanical ventilation.

Training in the Use of a Ventilator If the use of ventilators is part of your scope of practice, you should get training in ventilator management and mechanical ventilation.

Participate in high-fidelity simulation exercises that are designed to imitate different breathing and airway conditions as part of your training for simulations. This kind of practical experience is essential for the growth of one's abilities.

CPR and BLS Renewal: It is imperative that you remain current with the recommendations for cardiopulmonary resuscitation (CPR) and basic life support (BLS), as these abilities are necessary in the event of an emergency involving the airway or breathing.

Collaborative Respiratory Therapy Work With Respiratory Therapists To Gain Insight Into More Advanced Respiratory Assessment And Treatment Methods Collaborate with respiratory therapists.

Cardiology is covered in Chapter 7.

The evaluation and treatment of cardiac disorders as well as cardiac emergencies are included in cardiology, which is an essential part of the field of paramedicine. Knowing how the circulatory system works, being able to identify cardiac problems, and being able to provide appropriate treatment are all necessary abilities for paramedics. In this chapter, we will investigate the structure of the heart, as well as cardiac evaluation, common cardiac disorders, and the therapies that paramedics use to treat cardiac emergencies.

The Internal Structure of the Heart

The heart is a muscular organ that is responsible for pumping oxygenated blood to the tissues and organs of the body, while at the same time receiving deoxygenated blood from these places so that it can be oxygenated in the lungs. This process is called cardiopulmonary exchange. When it comes to diagnosing and treating cardiac diseases, having a solid understanding of the architecture of the heart is absolutely necessary.

The Various Parts of the Heart:

There are four chambers in the heart, and each of these chambers performs a distinct function during the cardiac cycle.

The right atrium is responsible for pumping deoxygenated blood into the right ventricle after receiving it from the body.

The right ventricle is the chamber of the heart that receives blood from the right atrium and then pumps that blood to the lungs so that it can be oxygenated.

The left atrium is responsible for pumping oxygenated blood into the left ventricle after receiving it from the lungs.

Left Ventricle: This chamber is responsible for receiving blood from the left atrium, pumping the blood into the systemic circulation, and providing oxygen to the various tissues throughout the body.

Valves that:

There are four valves in the heart that prevent blood from flowing backwards through the chambers:

The tricuspid valve is a one-way valve that stops blood from flowing backwards into the right atrium. It is located between the right ventricle and the right atrium.

Pulmonary Valve: This valve is located at the beginning of the pulmonary artery, and it is responsible for separating the right ventricle from the pulmonary circulation.

The mitral valve, also known as the bicuspid valve, is situated between the left atrium and the left ventricle. Its job is to stop the flow of blood from the left ventricle back into the left atrium.

The left ventricle and the rest of the cardiovascular system are kept apart by the aortic valve, which is located near the beginning of the aorta.

Donation of Blood:

The coronary arteries are responsible for supplying oxygenated blood to the heart at all times, which is a requirement of the heart itself. The following are the two primary coronary arteries:

The Right Coronary Artery, also known as the RCA, is the blood vessel that nourishes the right atrium, the right ventricle, and a section of the interventricular septum.

The Left Main Coronary Artery is the one that splits into the Left Anterior Descending Artery (LAD) and the Left Circumflex Artery (LCx). While the LCx artery provides blood to the left atrium and the posterior portion of the left ventricle, the LAD artery is responsible for supplying the anterior portion of the left ventricle as well as the interventricular septum.

Electrification Method:

The electrical system of the heart is responsible for controlling the rhythm as well as the coordination of its contractions. The electrical impulse begins in the sinoatrial (SA) node, sometimes known as the "natural pacemaker," and then moves via the atria and the atrioventricular (AV) node before reaching the ventricles. The SA node is responsible for initiating the electrical impulse. The atrial and ventricular contractions in the heart become synchronized as a result of this process.

Evaluation of the Heart

An evaluation of a patient's cardiac health is referred to as a cardiac assessment. The major objective of a cardiac assessment is to recognize the signs and symptoms of cardiac problems or emergent situations in a patient. The following are important parts of a cardiac assessment:

Obtaining a Comprehensive Patient History It is important to obtain a complete patient history, which should include information on chest pain or discomfort, past cardiac events, risk factors (such as smoking, family history, and hypertension), and current medications.

Patient Presentation: Pay attention to the patient's overall look, taking note of any indicators of discomfort such as paleness, diaphoresis (excessive sweating), or odd postures.

Measurements of Vital Signs: Be sure to take measurements of your vital signs, including your heart rate, blood pressure, breathing rate, and oxygen saturation. Variations in these parameters can provide useful information about the patient's cardiac health.

Examine the patient's chest, listen to their heart sounds, check for peripheral edema, and listen to their jugular venous distention (JVD) and lung sounds. Conduct a focused physical examination.

12-Lead ECG: It is important to obtain a 12-lead electrocardiogram (ECG) in order to evaluate the electrical activity of the heart and diagnose any arrhythmias, ischemia, or infarctions that may be present.

Cardiac Biomarkers: Evaluate cardiac biomarkers to test for myocardial injury, particularly in the context of chest pain. Some examples of cardiac biomarkers include troponin and creatine kinase-MB (CK-MB).

Conditions of the Heart That Are Frequently Seen Along with Emergencies

A wide variety of heart problems and emergent situations are something that paramedics see on a regular basis. The following are some of the most frequent:

Myocardial Infarction (also known as a Heart Attack): A myocardial infarction, also known as a heart attack, happens when there is a blockage in the coronary arteries, which results in the heart muscle not receiving enough blood flow. It manifests with chest discomfort that is strong and crushing, and it frequently radiates to the left arm, the neck, or the jaw. Aspirin and nitroglycerin are given by paramedics, and if oxygen is required, the paramedics also hasten the patient's transport to a facility that is competent of performing percutaneous coronary intervention (PCI).

Angina Pectoris: Angina is a condition that causes pain or discomfort in the chest and is caused by temporary ischemia of the myocardium. Exertion is the most common trigger for this condition, and rest or nitroglycerin are the most effective treatments. Nitroglycerin is given to the patient, and they are monitored by the paramedics.

Arrhythmias are a type of aberrant cardiac rhythm that can range from being completely harmless to being a potentially fatal condition. After determining the type of arrhythmia, emergency medical technicians may treat the patient with medicine, a defibrillator, or synchronized cardioversion, depending on the circumstances.

Heart Failure is a condition in which the heart is unable to pump blood adequately and is hence referred to as failing to pump the heart. Dyspnea, sometimes known as shortness of breath, is one of the symptoms, along with fatigue and peripheral edema. It's possible that paramedics will give patients medication, oxygen, and conduct an assessment to look for potential explanations of the worsening condition.

Cardiogenic Shock: Cardiogenic shock is a severe kind of heart failure in which the heart is unable to pump enough blood to fulfill the demands of the body. This results in the patient going into cardiac arrest. It is an extremely urgent situation that calls for advanced cardiac procedures and possibly even support for the circulation.

Aortic Dissection An aortic dissection is a disorder that can be fatal and is defined by a tear in the aortic wall. This tear allows blood to enter the aorta and separates the layers of the aorta. Controlling the patient's blood pressure and getting them to a surgical center as quickly as possible are two of the primary responsibilities of paramedics.

The term "cardiac arrest" refers to the condition that happens when the heart suddenly stops beating normally. The emergency medical technicians begin cardiopulmonary resuscitation (CPR) and utilize automated external defibrillators (AEDs) in an effort to return the patient's heart rhythm to a normal pattern.

Congestive Heart Failure: Congestive heart failure is a chronic disorder in which the heart is unable to pump blood effectively, resulting to fluid accumulation in the lungs and peripheral tissues. This condition is characterized by a progressive worsening of symptoms over time. The management of symptoms, the distribution of drugs, and the provision of oxygen are all tasks performed by paramedics.

Interventions for the Heart

In the management of cardiac diseases and crises, the provision of measures to stabilize the patient's condition and reduce the risk of additional injury is an important part of the role that paramedics play. The following are some of the most important cardiac interventions that paramedics perform:

Oxygen Therapy entails the administration of supplementary oxygen in order to keep adequate oxygen saturation levels. These levels are essential for the functioning of the heart and brain.

Patients who are suspected of having a myocardial infarction (also known as a heart attack) should be given aspirin in order to inhibit platelet aggregation and decrease the creation of further clots.

Nitroglycerin: Nitroglycerin should be given to the patient in order to alleviate chest pain (angina) and to enhance blood flow to the heart.

Defibrillation: In cases of ventricular fibrillation or pulseless ventricular tachycardia, automated external defibrillators (AEDs) should be used to deliver electrical shocks to the heart in order to defibrillate the patient.

Patients diagnosed with certain types of tachyarrhythmias may benefit from having synchronized cardioversion procedures performed in order to achieve a return to a normal rhythm in their hearts.

Medication Administer a wide variety of medications to the patient, such as antiarrhythmics, vasodilators, inotropes, and analgesics, depending on how the patient's condition requires them to be used.

ECG with 12 Leads: Carry out ECGs with 12 leads to evaluate the electrical activity of the heart and diagnose a variety of cardiac problems.

High-Performance CPR In the event that someone has cardiac arrest, it is imperative that they get high-quality cardiopulmonary resuscitation (CPR) immediately.

During a cardiac emergency, it is imperative to check and make sure that the patient has a clear airway in order to maintain oxygenation and ventilation.

Care Following a Heart Attack

After the first treatment for cardiac problems, it is the responsibility of the paramedics to continue monitoring the patient's health and to make sure that the handoff of care to the receiving facility goes as smoothly as possible. These are the following:

During travel, it is imperative that the vital signs, electrocardiogram (ECG), and overall clinical state of the patient be continuously monitored and evaluated.

Administer drugs to the patient as directed by the doctor and keep track of how the patient reacts to each medication.

Maintain communication with the facility that will be receiving the patient by providing vital patient information such as the patient's medical history, the interventions that were performed, and the patient's response to therapy.

Reassessment: It is important to conduct reassessments on a regular basis in order to detect any shifts in the patient's state and to modify treatment accordingly.

Case Studies: Practical Aspects of Cardiology

Consider the following case studies to illustrate how the theory of cardiology might be applied practically in the field of paramedicine:

ST-Elevation Myocardial Infarction (STEMI) is the topic of the first case study.

You are dispatched to assist a male patient aged 56 who is complaining of significant chest pain that is radiating to his left arm. You discover the patient to be in extreme distress, sweating heavily, and gripping his chest when you arrive at the scene. You swiftly examine his vital signs and carry out a 12-lead electrocardiogram, which confirms that the ST-segment elevation is present in the patient's anterior leads. This is very suggestive of an ST-elevation myocardial infarction (STEMI), which stands for ST-elevation myocardial infarction. You start high-performance CPR as soon as possible, provide aspirin and nitroglycerin as soon as possible, and go as quickly as possible to a facility that is equipped to perform cardiac catheterization and intervention in an emergency situation.

Case Study No. 2: Tachycardia of the Ventricles

You are on your way to a patient's home when you receive a call that they are feeling chest pain along with palpitations. During the assessment, you see that the patient is awake and has good blood flow, but they have a pulse that is erratic and an electrocardiogram rhythm that indicates they have ventricular tachycardia (VT). You make hasty preparations to get the defibrillator ready for a possible cardioversion. In an effort to return the heart to its normal sinus rhythm, you give the patient an antiarrhythmic medicine such as amiodarone and then attempt synchronized cardioversion. You continue to evaluate the patient's response while providing the proper post-cardioversion treatment while the rhythm of the patient's heart changes to sinus.

Exacerbation of Congestive Heart Failure is Examined in Case Study No. 3

You get a call about a woman who is 68 years old and has a history of congestive heart failure (CHF). She is complaining of increased shortness of breath and peripheral edema when you get at the scene. As soon as you arrive, you see that the patient is experiencing significant respiratory distress, and a lung auscultation reveals bilateral crackles. You give the patient oxygen, check their vital signs, and give them nitroglycerin in the hopes that it may relieve their angina. You also give the patient intravenous diuretics in order to lower their fluid overload, and you carefully watch how they react to the medication. You are going to transport the patient to a facility that specializes in cardiac care so that they can undergo further examination and treatment.

Education on Going in the Field of Cardiology

It is important for paramedics to participate in continual education and training in order to keep up with the most recent advancements in cardiology. Continuing education opportunities in cardiology can be found in the following places:

Advanced Cardiac Life Support (ACLS): ACLS courses offer in-depth instruction on the management of cardiac emergencies, including advanced arrhythmia diagnosis and treatment. These courses can be found online.

12-Lead ECG Interpretation: Taking advanced classes in 12-lead ECG interpretation enables paramedics to better recognize and diagnose a variety of heart problems.

Participate in high-fidelity simulation exercises that simulate cardiac settings so that you may get some hands-on experience. This is part of the training for simulation.

Review of Cases: In this activity, you will work with your coworkers to discuss hard cardiac cases and provide your opinions on various treatment techniques.

Attending Cardiology Conferences and Workshops It is important to keep up with the latest developments in the field of cardiology, hence it is beneficial to attend cardiology conferences and workshops.

Accessing Online Resources To keep up to speed with the most recent cardiology guidelines and research, it is important to utilize online resources. Some examples of these tools are webinars, forums, and medical journals.

The Trauma Chapter (Chapter 8)

The evaluation and treatment of injuries sustained as a result of traumatic events such as accidents, falls, acts of violence, and other traumatic occurrences are the primary focuses of trauma care in the field of paramedicine. When it comes to delivering prompt medical attention to trauma patients and ensuring that they are given the right treatment while being transported to the hospital, paramedics play a pivotal role. In this chapter, we will discuss the fundamentals of trauma evaluation, the various ways in which traumatic injuries can be categorized, as well as the strategies and treatments that paramedics use in emergency situations involving trauma patients.

Assessment of Trauma: Foundational Principles

Patients who have been injured are subjected to a comprehensive evaluation as part of the trauma assessment process. This evaluation is typically geared toward the detection of life-threatening conditions that call for prompt medical attention. The following are important aspects of a trauma assessment:

Safety at the site: It is imperative that you, your crew, and the patient all remain safe while at the site. Find any potential dangers, such as downed electrical lines or unsafe structures, and take measures to eliminate them.

Gathering information on the incident that led to the injury is vital because it might provide important clues regarding the nature and severity of the trauma. The mechanism of the injury is the event that led to the injury.

Patient Presentation: Take note of the patient's general appearance, paying particular attention to any indicators of discomfort, degree of awareness, and vital signs. Take careful note of any signs of trauma, such as blood or deformities in the patient.

Primary Survey: To identify and treat potentially life-threatening conditions, do a primary survey as quickly as possible. Assessing the patient's airway, breathing, and circulation (abbreviated as ABC) and resolving concerns in this order are required to carry out this procedure.

The first step in performing an airway assessment is to ensure that the airway is clear of any impediments. Make sure the patient is in the correct posture, and employ airway maneuvers to open their airway if necessary.

Evaluation of Breathing Determine whether or not the patient is breathing adequately while looking for indicators of respiratory distress or failure. Take care of any problems, such as chest trauma, that might be affecting your ability to breathe.

Evaluation of the Circulation To evaluate the circulation, first determine whether or not peripheral pulses are present and evaluate their quality. Take care of any bleeding that is visible on the surface of the body, and evaluate whether or not intravenous (IV) access and fluid resuscitation are necessary.

Use the Glasgow Coma Scale (GCS) to evaluate the patient's state of consciousness and neurological function. This assists in the evaluation of brain injury as well as the identification of changes in mental status.

Control of the Patient's Environment and Exposure Expose the patient in order to check for injuries and keep their body temperature stable. If it becomes necessary, take precautions against hypothermia.

Secondary Survey: Carry out a thorough secondary survey in order to evaluate whether or not there are any more injuries that are not immediately life-threatening. This comprises a complete examination from head to toe as well as radiographic studies if they are available.

Documentation: Make sure to document your activities and results, including recording vital signs, injuries, patient history, and any interventions that were carried out.

A Breakdown of the Different Types of Traumatic Injuries

The nature and severity of traumatic injuries might vary greatly from case to case. A classification system is utilized by paramedics in order to appropriately categorize trauma patients and establish the necessary level of care. The Mechanism, Anatomic Injury, Physiological Abnormality, and Comorbid Conditions (MAP-IT) method is the type of classification that is utilized the vast majority of the time.

The action or series of events that led to the trauma is referred to as the mechanism of the injury. Injuries caused by common methods include falling, being involved in a car accident, being shot, being stabbed, or being crushed. Accidents involving motor vehicles that are traveling at high speeds or falls from substantial heights are examples of high-energy processes that are more likely to result in serious injuries.

Injuries Sustained by the Patient Specific injuries suffered by the patient are referred to as the patient's anatomic injuries. The head, neck, chest, belly, and pelvis are some of the body parts that are used to classify these injuries. Other categories include the extremities. The severity can range from relatively small contusions and abrasions to more serious fractures, dislocations, organ damage, or even amputations.

Abnormalities of the Patient's Physiology Physiological abnormalities relate to the patient's vital signs and their general condition. The patient's airway, breathing, circulation, and other vital signs, as well as their GCS score, are all evaluated by the paramedics. The presence of abnormal findings may point to a critical situation such as shock, hypoxia, brain injury, or another ailment.

Comorbid Conditions: Comorbid conditions are any pre-existing medical conditions that may make it more difficult for a patient to recover from a traumatic event. Diabetes, hypertension, bleeding disorders, and the usage of anticoagulants are all potential examples of these ailments.

By making use of the MAP-IT system, paramedics are able to rapidly evaluate the patient's overall status and adapt their treatment strategies accordingly. For instance, a patient who has been shot in the chest and is exhibiting indications of shock might need to be rushed to a trauma center as soon as possible so that they can have emergency surgery.

Various Interventions for Trauma

In order to stabilize trauma patients and protect them from further injury, paramedics receive extensive training in a variety of lifesaving techniques. The specific interventions are determined by the injuries sustained by the patient as well as their clinical presentation. The following are examples of common trauma interventions:

Controlling the Hemorrhage Direct pressure, hemostatic agents, tourniquets (as a last resort), and pressure dressings are all effective methods for controlling external bleeding. Internal bleeding may necessitate access to an IV and the administration of fluid resuscitation.

Airway Management: Ensure that the patient has a patent airway by utilizing the proper maneuvers, adjuncts (such as oropharyngeal or nasopharyngeal airways), and, if necessary, advanced airway management techniques such as endotracheal intubation.

Assisting with breathing by means of bag-valve-mask (BVM) ventilation or mechanical ventilators is what is meant by "breathing support." Chest decompression could be necessary in cases where chest injuries are suspected.

Support of Circulation: Restore circulation by evaluating for hypovolemic shock and treating it with fluids administered intravenously (IV) if it is needed. In the event of a massive loss of blood, blood products should be given.

Immobilization of the Cervical Spine: In order to prevent injuries to the spinal cord, it is important to stabilize the cervical spine. This could involve manually immobilizing the patient or applying cervical collars to the patient.

Immobilization of fractures and dislocations using splints or traction devices is the first step in the fracture and dislocation management process. When it is absolutely required, administer pain relief.

Pain Management: Administer analgesics to the patient in order to lessen the patient's discomfort and to lower the patient's anxiety level.

Care for Wounds Make sure any open wounds, lacerations, or burns are cleaned and dressed properly to lower the chance of infection and further harm to the tissue.

Burn Management Take care of burns caused by heat, chemicals, or electricity in accordance with predetermined procedures for burns. Determine what proportion of the patient's total body surface area is impacted before beginning resuscitation efforts.

Immobilization of the Spine In the event that a spinal injury is suspected, appropriate immobilization with spine boards and cervical collars must be performed.

Pelvic Binders: When treating suspected pelvic fractures and attempting to control bleeding, pelvic binders or stabilizers may be utilized.

Preparation for Transport: In order to prepare the patient for transport to the hospital, it may be necessary to secure them to a backboard or stretcher, and it is important to check their vital signs while they are being transported.

Concerning Trauma, Special Considerations

Certain types of catastrophic injuries and patient demographics need for further care and treatment, including the following:

Patients who have had head trauma may have elevated levels of intracranial pressure, abbreviated as ICP. In order to prevent hypoxia, paramedics need to ensure that appropriate ventilation and oxygenation are being provided, and they should also avoid hyperventilation, which can make intracranial pressure (ICP) worse.

Patients who have suffered pediatric trauma have distinctive physiological responses to the injuries they sustained. It is necessary for paramedics to be skilled in evaluating and treating children, taking into account the unique requirements and anatomical peculiarities of younger patients.

Trauma in the elderly can be complicated by the presence of preexisting medical disorders; as a result, elderly people are more likely to suffer fractures and brain injuries. When treating patients' pain, paramedics need to exercise caution and keep potential drug interactions in mind.

Patients Who Are Pregnant: The management of trauma in pregnant patients involves a special set of concerns. Assessing for suspected fetal distress, putting the ABCs in priority order, and using the left lateral tilt to relieve inferior vena cava compression are all things that paramedics should do.

Some trauma patients have injuries that affect many body systems, and this condition is referred to as multi-system trauma. Interventions provided by paramedics have to be prioritized according to the severity of the patient's condition.

Patients who have experienced either drowning or coming dangerously close to drowning require airway care and oxygenation. The risk of hypothermia should likewise not be discounted.

Case Studies: Different Types of Disasters

Consider the following case studies as illustrations of how trauma assessment and therapies might be practically applied in real life situations:

Case Study 1: Accident Involving a Motor Vehicle (MVA)

You have arrived at the site of a car accident that involved a head-on collision between two vehicles. One of the drivers is helpless inside their vehicle, while the other is unable to communicate with them. A major mechanism of injury, a decreased level of awareness, and shallow breathing are some of the findings of the fast assessment that you perform on the patient. After removing the patient from the dangerous situation, you will intubate their endotracheal tube to protect their airway, create an IV access point, and give them IV fluids. The patient's Glasgow Coma Scale (GCS) score is still very low, and you are continuously monitoring their condition while rushing them to a trauma hospital.

Fall from a Great Height (Case Study No. 2)

You are dispatched to the scene of an accident involving a construction worker who has fallen off of a scaffolding. The patient is found lying on the ground with many fractures, including an open fracture to the femur, as well as evidence of extensive external bleeding when you arrive. You use direct pressure and bandages to stop the bleeding, stabilize the broken femur, and administer pain medication in order to treat the patient. A subsequent search confirms that there are no further injuries that are life-threatening. While you are doing so, you bring the patient to the closest hospital and continue to keep close monitoring on them.

Case Study 3: An Instance of Stabbing

You are dispatched to a patient's home who has a stab wound to the chest and needs immediate medical attention. During the exam, you notice that the patient is suffering from significant respiratory distress, and you also notice that there is a knife imbedded in the patient's chest. In a short amount of time, you apply an occlusive dressing to the wound in order to prevent infection, assist with ventilations, set up an IV access point, and get ready for emergency transport. As the patient's condition worsens during transport, you conduct a needle decompression to relieve tension pneumothorax. This allows the patient to breathe easier. As soon as they got to the hospital, the surgical team got to work on the patient's injury right away.

Continuing Education in Acute Stress Disorder

It is important for paramedics to participate in continual education and training in order to keep up with the most recent advancements in trauma care. The following are some options for furthering one's education in the field of trauma:

Advanced Trauma Life Support (ATLS): Advanced Trauma Life Support (ATLS) courses offer in-depth training on the evaluation and management of trauma patients, with a particular emphasis on critical decision-making.

Prehospital Trauma Life Support (PHTLS): Prehospital Trauma Life Support (PHTLS) courses are designed to explicitly address prehospital trauma care and cover assessment, interventions, and transfer of trauma patients.

Participate in high-fidelity simulation exercises that imitate traumatic circumstances and provide hands-on practice. This type of training is known as simulation training.

Participating in Trauma-Related Conferences and Workshops It is important to keep up with the most recent developments in trauma care by participating in trauma-related conferences and workshops.

Classes on Bleeding Control: Learn how to apply tourniquets, pack wounds, and use hemostatic agents, among other strategies for controlling bleeding.

Radiographic Interpretation: Sharpen your skills in identifying traumatic injuries using X-rays and other types of radiographic examinations by improving your ability to do radiographic interpretation.

Emergencies of a Medical Nature, Chapter 9

Emergencies in the field of medicine can refer to a wide variety of diseases and ailments, ranging from difficulties breathing and heart problems to neurological abnormalities and metabolic imbalances. In these kinds of emergencies, paramedics are frequently the first people to arrive on the scene. This means that they need the knowledge and abilities necessary to evaluate patients' severe medical conditions and give them with prompt care. In this chapter, we will discuss the fundamentals of medical evaluation, common medical emergencies, and the interventions and treatments that paramedics use to treat and manage these types of situations.

Fundamentals of the Medical Examining Process

The evaluation of medical emergencies entails doing a comprehensive assessment of patients who present themselves with acute medical issues. This procedure seeks to discover issues that could potentially endanger life and direct necessary interventions. The following are important parts of a medical assessment:

Safety at the site: It is imperative that both the patient and the responders be kept safe while at the site. Determine the potential risks and take measures to reduce them.

Collecting information on the beginning and progression of the illness, as well as the patient's past medical history and drug use, is an important step in determining the disease's mechanism.

Patient Presentation: Pay attention to the patient's overall look, making mental status assessments, noting any indicators of discomfort, and taking the patient's vital signs.

Primary Survey: To identify and treat potentially life-threatening conditions, do a primary survey as quickly as possible. The airway, breathing, and circulation of the patient should be the primary concerns, and difficulties should be addressed in this sequence.

Assessing the Airway In this step, you will evaluate how clear the airway is and look for any obstructions. Make sure the patient is in the correct posture, and employ airway maneuvers to open their airway if necessary.

Evaluation of Breathing Determine whether or not the patient is breathing adequately while looking for indicators of respiratory distress or failure. Take care of concerns such as compromised respiratory function, chest pain, and altered mental condition.

Evaluation of the Circulation To evaluate the circulation, first determine whether or not peripheral pulses are present and evaluate their quality. As directed, drugs should be administered, and supportive care should be provided.

Disability: Using instruments like the Glasgow Coma Scale (GCS), determine the patient's state of neurological consciousness. This assists in evaluating the patient's altered mental status as well as any neurological problems.

Exposure and Environment Control: Expose the patient to determine whether or not they have any medical conditions or concerns, and make sure that their body temperature is maintained. If it becomes necessary, take precautions against hypothermia.

Conduct a thorough secondary survey by conducting an examination of the patient from head to toe and acquiring a patient history in order to uncover any further medical problems.

Documentation Be sure to keep a record of all of your discoveries and activities, including vital signs, symptoms, and any treatments or interventions you administer. Maintaining a consistent level of treatment requires accurate documentation at all times.

Frequent instances of medical urgency

Because of the diversity of the medical crises they respond to, paramedics must adjust their methods of assessment and treatment to each individual patient. The following are examples of common medical emergencies:

Patients may come with a variety of respiratory issues, including asthma, chronic obstructive pulmonary disease (COPD), pulmonary edema, or anaphylaxis. Respiratory Distress and Failure: Patients may present with a number of respiratory disorders. When it is necessary, paramedics will supply oxygen, administer bronchodilators, and provide support for ventilation.

Convulsions: Convulsions can be the outcome of a number of different medical disorders, such as epilepsy or underlying infections. The provision of breathing support and the administration of drugs to manage seizures are all part of the paramedic's job description.

Patients with diabetes are at risk for experiencing diabetic emergencies, which include hypoglycemia (low blood sugar) and hyperglycemia (high blood sugar), all of which require the administration of glucose or insulin, respectively.

Reactions to Allergic Substances: Anaphylaxis can be caused by allergic reactions to substances such as meals, drugs, or the stings of insects. In order to ease symptoms, paramedics will typically deliver epinephrine, antihistamines, and steroids.

Ischemic strokes are those that are caused by blood clots, and hemorrhagic strokes are those that are caused by bleeding in the brain. The symptoms of a stroke are quickly identified by paramedics, who then expeditiously take the patient to a facility that is able to deliver clot-busting drugs.

Sepsis is a systemic inflammatory response that can occur as a result of an infection. The probable indicators of sepsis are identified by paramedics, who also assist with oxygenation, set up intravenous access, and deliver fluids, antibiotics, and other treatments.

Changes in Mental Status Patients who present with changes in their mental status may have underlying causes such as head trauma, drunkenness, or metabolic problems. Assessing and treating the underlying problem while also providing supportive care is what paramedics do.

Pain in the Chest Pain in the chest can be caused by a number of different things, including problems with the heart (such as angina or a myocardial infarction), musculoskeletal pain, or gastrointestinal disorders. Assessing for symptoms of myocardial ischemia and providing treatment accordingly are two of the tasks performed by paramedics.

Syncope, often known as passing out, can be brought on by a number of different things, including vasovagal episodes or underlying heart problems. Assessing the situation and treating the underlying problem while maintaining adequate oxygenation is the job of paramedics.

Interventions from the Medical Field

The training that paramedics get prepares them to stabilize patients experiencing a variety of medical crises using a variety of treatment modalities. The patient's state and the underlying medical issue both play a role in the specific interventions that are used. The following are examples of common medical interventions:

Management of the Airway Ensure that the patient has a patent airway by employing the proper maneuvers and adjuncts (such as oropharyngeal or nasopharyngeal airways). It is possible that more advanced methods of airway control, such as endotracheal intubation, will be required.

Assisting with breathing by means of bag-valve-mask (BVM) ventilation or mechanical ventilators is what is meant by "breathing support." Take care of any underlying respiratory problems, such as bronchospasm, and make sure oxygenation is adequate.

Monitoring of the Heart The monitoring of the heart's rhythms using electrocardiography (ECG) to look for arrhythmias or ischemic abnormalities is known as cardiac monitoring.

Administration of Medication It is necessary to administer medications to the patient according on their condition. These medications may include analgesics, antiarrhythmics, bronchodilators, and anticonvulsants.

IV Access: It is important to create an intravenous (IV) access in order to administer drugs and fluids, particularly in circumstances where the patient is hypotensive or dehydrated.

Management of Glucose Patients who have diabetes or altered mental status as a result of metabolic disorders should have glucose or insulin administered in order to maintain their blood sugar levels.

Pain management involves administering analgesics in order to reduce the patient's perception of pain and increase their level of comfort.

Medication Administered Through the Nasal Route In the event that the patient is experiencing seizures or cardiac problems, certain medications should be given through the nasal route so that they can be absorbed quickly.

Intramuscular medicine Administration When intravenous access is not easily available, intramuscular medicine administration is the next best option.

In the Event of a Medical Emergency, Special Considerations

Certain types of medical situations and patient demographics call for more care and attention, including the following:

Acute myocardial infarction (AMI): It is critical to recognize the symptoms of AMI as quickly as possible and analyze the situation for possible interventions. Aspirin, nitroglycerin, and analgesics are among possible treatments that paramedics can provide.

Patients who are pregnant: Certain pregnancy-related conditions, such as preeclampsia and eclampsia, may call for particular medical attention. Assessing and treating these disorders is a skill that paramedics need to be adept in.

Patients of All Ages Because of their distinct physiological reactions to a variety of medical conditions, pediatric patients and patients of all ages who are considered geriatric patients require specialized assessment and treatment skills from paramedics.

Emergencies of a Psychiatric Nature It is possible for paramedics to come across patients who are undergoing acute psychiatric crises. It is crucial for their safety to engage in careful examination as well as communication.

In the event of a neurologic emergency, prompt recognition of symptoms such as a stroke or a change in mental state is essential. When dealing with patients suffering from these illnesses, paramedics are required to adhere to certain guidelines.

Case Studies: Real-World Examples of Medical Emergencies

Consider the following case studies to illustrate how the theoretical concepts of medical assessment and intervention might be put into practice:

Case Study No. 1: A Severe Exacerbation of Asthma

After receiving a call about a woman in her 28th year who is having serious difficulty breathing and wheezing, you go to check on her. Upon arriving, you discover the patient in a tripod position, and they are using their auxiliary muscles in addition to wheezing audibly. The readout from her pulse oximeter is 88%. You start high-flow oxygen, provide albuterol using a nebulizer, and establish IV access in preparation for the possible introduction of corticosteroids. You continue to monitor the patient and provide supportive treatment as they are being transported to the hospital, and the patient's respiratory condition begins to improve.

Case Study 2: Hypoglycemia in Patients with Diabetes

You are dispatched to the location of a man who is 56 years old and has an altered mental status. Upon examination, the patient was found to be sweating excessively and to be confused. A value of 45 mg/dL was obtained for their blood glucose level. You give the patient glucose by mouth, and they experience a quick improvement in their mental status. You take the patient to the hospital so that further examination and treatment can be administered there.

Case Study No. 3: Possible Stroke Victim

You have been sent to the home of a 68-year-old male who has suddenly developed left-sided weakness and slurred speech. During the assessment, you see that the patient has a sagging face, hemiparesis on the left side of their body, and trouble speaking. Rapidly assessing the patient's vital signs, performing an evaluation using the Cincinnati Prehospital Stroke Scale, and transporting the patient to a stroke center in order to receive possible clot-busting drugs and advanced care are all things that you do.

Education on Going for Emergencies in the Medical Field

It is important for paramedics to participate in continual education and training in order to keep up with the most recent advances in the treatment of medical emergencies. The following are some options for furthering one's education in the field of emergency medical care:

Advanced Medical Life Support (AMLS): Courses in AMLS include in-depth instruction on the assessment and management of a variety of medical disorders, including advanced airway management and cardiac emergencies.

PALS stands for Pediatric Advanced Life Support. PALS courses focus especially on the care of pediatric patients and encompass pediatric assessment as well as the management of a variety of pediatric emergencies.

Geriatric Education for Emergency Medical Services (GEMS): GEMS courses place an emphasis on the distinct medical requirements and evaluation of older persons.

Participate in high-fidelity simulation exercises that provide hands-on practice and simulate various medical scenarios. This type of training is called simulation training.

Participate in Medical Conferences and Workshops It is important to participate in medical conferences and workshops so that you can learn about the most recent developments in medical emergency treatment.

Stay up to date with the latest modifications in drug protocols and new pharmacological therapies for medical disorders with the "Pharmacology Updates."

Obstetrics and Pediatrics are Covered in Chapter 10

Both obstetrics and pediatrics are sub-fields of paramedicine that focus specifically on the requirements that pregnant patients and young patients have that differ from those of adults. When it comes to providing treatment for expecting moms, newborns, and pediatric patients, paramedics play a very important role. In this chapter, we will discuss the fundamentals of obstetric and pediatric assessment, as well as prevalent diseases and complications, as well as the interventions and treatments that paramedics use for these particular patient populations.

Evaluation and Treatment of the Obstetric Patient

Care for pregnant patients is the focus of obstetric paramedicine, which addresses issues ranging from prenatal problems to labor and delivery. It is necessary for paramedics to have an in-depth knowledge of pregnancy-related conditions, the phases of labor, and the process of giving birth. Among the most important aspects of obstetric examination and care are the following:

Complications During Pregnancy:

In the course of their work, paramedics may come across pregnant patients who are suffering from hypertensive disorders such as preeclampsia or gestational hypertension. It is crucial to keep an eye on the patient's blood pressure and look for warning symptoms of severe preeclampsia.

Bleeding from the Vagina It is important to check for bleeding from the vagina, which can have a variety of causes including placental previa or abruption.

Recognize the indicators of preterm labor, like as contractions and changes in the cervical cervix, and consider using tocolytic drugs to suppress labor if you have any of these symptoms.

Multiple Gestation: It is extremely important to identify multiple pregnancies (such as twins or triplets), as these pregnancies pose higher dangers than single pregnancies do.

Ruptured Membranes: Determine whether or whether the patient's membranes have ruptured, then evaluate the patient for the possibility of any consequences.

Progress through Labor:

First Stage: It is important to be aware of the first stage of labor, which consists of contractions as well as a dilated cervix. In the event that labor is near, provide support for pain management measures and transport the patient to a facility that offers obstetric services.

The second stage of labor, often known as delivery, occurs after the first stage. Make preparations for an emergency birth and be ready to provide newborn resuscitation in case it's required.

In the third stage, which occurs after the birth of the infant, an examination for symptoms of placental delivery and separation is performed.

Evaluation and Care for Newborn Infants

Apgar Score It is important to determine the newborn's Apgar score in order to evaluate their general state and determine whether or not they require resuscitation.

Temperature regulation requires that you make sure the newborn is kept warm in order to avoid hypothermia.

Care of the Umbilical chord In order to properly care for the umbilical chord, first check for any bleeding or other complications.

Obstacles During Labor and Delivery:

Shoulder dystocia: During delivery, it is important to recognize and manage shoulder dystocia.

Postpartum Hemorrhage: Conduct a postpartum hemorrhage assessment and take the proper actions to reduce bleeding if one is found.

Neonatal Resuscitation: You should do neonatal resuscitation whenever it is necessary. This includes taking care of the airway and providing ventilation.

Pediatric Evaluation and Medical Attention

To be able to evaluate and provide care for children of all ages, ranging from infants to teenagers, one needs to have specialized training in pediatric paramedicine. Because of the distinctive physiological responses that children have to sickness and injury, it is vital for paramedics to modify their approach. Important aspects of pediatric evaluation and care include the following:

Evaluation Taking Into Account Age:

newborns: When caring for newborns, paramedics are required to take into consideration a variety of factors, including airway control and drug dosing.

Toddlers and Preschoolers: When evaluating and communicating with this age group, it is important to take into account their current stage of development as well as their communication abilities.

Children of School Age: To help minimize anxiety, provide explanations that are appropriate for their age group and involve these children in their care.

Respect the adolescents' right to autonomy as well as their right to privacy while including them in decision-making. Adolescents.

Conditions Relating to Children's Health:

Distress in the Respiratory Tract Croup, Asthma, and Bronchiolitis are just few of the illnesses that can cause pediatric patients to present with respiratory distress. Conduct an evaluation and administer any necessary interventions, such as bronchodilators.

Recognize and treat seizures in children, paying careful attention to the dosages of any medications they take and their overall safety.

Reactions to Allergens Take care of allergic reactions and give epinephrine as directed by the situation.

illnesses: Pediatric patients are more prone to illnesses such as febrile seizures or sepsis than patients of other ages. Examine the patient for any indications of infection and treat them as necessary.

Dehydration: Determine the severity of the dehydration in children and take the necessary steps to manage it, including administering the correct amount of fluids.

Injuries of a Traumatic Nature in Pediatrics:

Head Injuries: It is important to identify head injuries in children and conduct an evaluation to rule out the possibility of brain injury. Utilize assessment tools that are suitable for the patient's age, such as the Pediatric Glasgow Coma Scale.

Orthopedic Injuries: Treat fractures and dislocations in pediatric patients, paying particular attention to pain management and the application of the appropriate splints.

Injuries to the Abdomen It is important to screen children for abdominal damage and be aware of the indicators of internal injuries.

Taking Into Account Particulars:

Infant Airway: Have a solid understanding of how to manage an infant's airway, and take into consideration using a pediatric BVM that has a mask that is proportionate to the child's size.

Dosages: Determine the appropriate pediatric drug dosages based on the child's weight and then provide those dosages to the youngster.

Identifying Typical Developmental Milestones and Evaluating the Child's Growth and Development Level It is important to identify typical developmental milestones and evaluate the child's growth and development level.

Involvement of Parents and Caregivers It is important to involve parents and other caregivers in the assessment and care of their kid. In addition, parents should be provided with information and reassurance.

Emergencies That Are Common in Obstetrics and Pediatrics

Emergency medical technicians are regularly called upon to respond to obstetric and pediatric emergencies that call for prompt medical attention and action.

Emergencies Related to Pregnancy:

Recognize the symptoms of eclampsia, which is characterized by seizures in pregnant patients, and ensure that seizure control and speedy transport are provided.

Birth in Breech Position Determine whether or not the baby is in breech position during birth, and if this position is found, be prepared for any potential issues.

Umbilical Cord Prolapse: During delivery, it is important to manage any cases of umbilical cord prolapse in order to prevent cord compression.

Postpartum Hemorrhage: Postpartum hemorrhage can be controlled by administering medicine and doing fundal massage on the patient.

During delivery, it is important to be able to identify a prolapsed cord and take the right action to treat it.

Urgences Relating to Children:

Evaluation and management of febrile seizures in children, with the goals of guaranteeing the kid's safety and offering comfort to the child in the process.

Croup: Recognize croup, which is an infection of the upper airway caused by a virus, and give nebulized epinephrine if necessary.

Intussusception: Identify indicators of intussusception in newborns and examine for stomach pain and distension. Intussusception can be fatal.

Nebulized bronchodilators and corticosteroids, together with other medications, should be used to treat severe asthma attacks in children who have status asthmaticus.

Pediatric Cardiac Arrest: In the event of a pediatric cardiac arrest, do high-quality CPR on the child and employ defibrillation techniques that are appropriate for the child's age.

Various Methods of Intervention and Treatments

When caring for pediatric and obstetric patients, paramedics make use of a variety of procedures and treatments, including the following:

Interventions during Pregnancies:

Support during Labor: Offer physical and emotional support to laboring patients, as well as comfort measures.

Neonatal Resuscitation: It is important to do neonatal resuscitation and provide support throughout the transition to life outside of the uterus.

Postpartum Care: Assist with postpartum care, which includes evaluating the birth of the placenta and the mother's uterine contractions.

Medication Administration: In the case of preeclampsia, magnesium sulfate or oxytocin should be given. In the case of postpartum hemorrhage, oxytocin should be given.

Clinical Interventions for Children:

Airway Management Take care of the juvenile patient's airways utilizing approaches that are suitable for their age, such as bag-valve-mask ventilation and airway adjuncts.

Administering drugs: Administer drugs in accordance with pediatric dosages and methods, making sure to perform the appropriate calculations.

Establishing Intravenous Access It is important to establish intravenous access for pediatric patients when it is necessary. Smaller catheters should be used, and the kid should be monitored for signs of dehydration or shock.

Pain Management: Analgesics that are appropriate for the patient's age should be used to provide pain relief for pediatric patients.

Equipment Tailored to Your Needs:

Equipment Specific to Children Paramedics are equipped with equipment designed specifically for children, including oxygen masks, bag valve masks, and defibrillator pads sized specifically for children.

Availability of Obstetric Kits and Equipment It is imperative that obstetric kits and equipment be readily available for delivery.

The Practice of Obstetrics and Pediatrics Examined Through Case Studies

Consider the following case examples to illustrate how the theoretical concepts of obstetric and pediatric assessment and interventions might be put into practice:

Example 1: Labor That Began Too Soon

You get a call to assist a pregnant woman who is 32 years old and suffering regular contractions while she is 32 weeks along in her pregnancy. During the assessment, you notice that the patient is clearly experiencing pain, and you also observe contractions on the monitor. An examination of the cervical region reveals alterations. You begin the process of providing intravenous access, administer tocolytic drugs, provide oxygen, and transport the patient to a facility that offers obstetrical services. The objective is to postpone labor and give corticosteroids in order to promote healthy lung development in the fetus.

Case Study No. 2: Acute Respiratory Distress in Children

You have been sent to a house for a youngster who is experiencing difficulty breathing. The child is 4 years old. The youngster is seen to be sitting upright, making use of their auxiliary muscles, and exhibiting stridor when you arrive. You perform an assessment to look for possible causes, you know how to spot croup, and you give the patient nebulized epinephrine and corticosteroids. When the child's breathing becomes less labored, you rush them to the emergency room at the local hospital for further examination.

Case Study No. 3: A Postpartum Bleeding Complication

You are called to a postpartum patient who gave birth at home and is currently experiencing significant vaginal bleeding. As soon as you arrive, you begin an examination of the patient and look for indicators of postpartum hemorrhage. After doing fundal massage, administering uterotonics, establishing IV access, and transporting the patient to the hospital, you continue the patient's examination and consider whether or not surgical intervention is necessary.

Education Continued in the Fields of Obstetrics and Pediatrics

It is imperative that paramedics participate in continuous education and training in order to be abreast of the most recent advancements in obstetric and pediatric care. The following are some options for those interested in furthering their studies in these areas:

Care for Pregnant Women:

Advanced Obstetric Life Support (ALSO): Advanced Obstetric Life Support (ALSO) courses offer comprehensive instruction on the management of obstetric crises and deliveries.

Participate in high-fidelity obstetric simulations during your training to hone your skills in performing resuscitation on newborns and perfect your delivery procedures.

Concerning Children:

Pediatric Advanced Life Support (PALS): PALS courses focus on the assessment and management of pediatric crises, including advanced airway management and drug administration. PALS certification is required for medical professionals who work with children.

Participate in pediatric-specific simulation activities designed to recreate situations involving children of varying ages. This is referred to as "pediatric simulation."

Learn about developmental milestones and the specific components of pediatric care that are required for different age groups by reading about developmental pediatrics.

The Operations Chapter (Chapter 11)

The field of paramedicine is an evolving and intricate one, and the effectiveness of paramedic services is not only dependent on clinical understanding but also on efficient operations. In the following chapter, we will investigate the essential components of paramedic operations, which include emergency response systems, equipment and vehicles, communication, and quality improvement programs. It is vital to have an understanding of the operational side of paramedicine in order to provide patient care that is effective, safe, and of high quality.

Systems for Emergency and Disaster Response

The cornerstone of paramedicine is comprised of very effective emergency response systems. These systems consist of a number of different parts, such as emergency medical dispatch, response vehicles, and medical communications. Let's take a closer look at each of these individual components:

1. Emergency Medical Dispatch, abbreviated as "EMD"

People who are in need of assistance during a medical emergency should get in touch with emergency medical dispatch as their initial point of contact. EMDs go through extensive training that teaches them to prioritize replies, obtain information from callers, and provide pre-arrival instructions. The following are important EMD functions:

Screening of Calls Emergency management dispatchers (EMDs) screen incoming calls in order to establish the type and severity of an emergency and ensure that the right resources are deployed.

Instructions Prior to Arrival Emergency medical dispatchers (EMDs) give callers instructions prior to their arrival, such as CPR guidance, bleeding management, or delivery support.

Allocation of Resources Emergency medical dispatchers (EMDs) are responsible for assigning resources such as ambulances, paramedics, and people from the fire department based on the information that is acquired.

2. Vehicles for Emergency Response:

Many different types of response vehicles are used by paramedic services, and each one has a particular function. Because these cars are stocked with medical supplies and equipment, paramedics are able to give care both at the scene of the accident and while patients are being transported. The following are examples of common types of response vehicles:

Ambulances are the most common means by which patients are transported to medical institutions because they are pre-loaded with all of the necessary medical supplies.

Vehicles Providing Advanced Life Support (ALS): These ambulances are outfitted with the most cutting-edge medical technology and may also contain paramedics who are trained to carry out more complex medical operations.

BLS Vehicles, also known as Basic Life Support vehicles, are normally staffed with emergency medical technicians (EMTs) and are equipped with fundamental medical supplies.

Community Paramedicine Units: Certain ambulance services offer community paramedicine units, which are designed to deliver non-urgent medical care and support to patients in the comfort of their own homes or in other community settings.

3. Communications in the Medical Field:

In the field of paramedicine, effective communication is of the utmost importance. The coordination of care, the solicitation of more resources, and the transmission of patient information to healthcare facilities are all tasks that are dependent on various communication networks. The following are important aspects of medical communications:

Radio Systems: In order to communicate with dispatch, other first responders, and medical facilities, paramedics use radios that are capable of transmitting in both directions. It is essential to have proper radio etiquette in order to avoid misunderstandings and to guarantee that operations run smoothly.

Mobile Data Terminals (MDTs): MDTs give paramedics access to digital information, mapping, and patient data, which enables them to make informed decisions while they are on the scene of an emergency.

Telemedicine: Some ambulance services use telemedicine platforms to connect their paramedics with medical professionals, such as doctors and specialists, so that the paramedics can receive consultation and direction about patient care.

Vehicles and other forms of apparatus

In order to deliver care of the highest possible standard, paramedics use a diverse assortment of tools and vehicles. It is vital to be conversant with these tools and to do routine maintenance on them. Let's have a look at some of the most important aspects of the equipment and vehicles used in paramedicine:

1. Personal Protective Equipment, abbreviated as "PPE"

In order to protect themselves and others from infectious infections, paramedics use a variety of different types of personal protective equipment (PPE). Gloves, masks, gowns, and eye protection are all necessary pieces of personal protective equipment.

2. Surgical and Medical Equipment

The following are some examples of the kind of medical supplies that are typically found in paramedic vehicles:

Tools for Managing the Airway These tools include sophisticated airway devices such as endotracheal tubes and supraglottic airway devices in addition to airway adjuncts such as oropharyngeal and nasopharyngeal airways.

Monitoring Equipment for the Heart In order to evaluate patients' cardiac rhythms, provide defibrillation, and monitor patients while they are being transported, paramedics use electrocardiogram (ECG) monitors and defibrillators.

IV Supplies: When an IV access point has been established, paramedics are able to provide fluids and medications more effectively. This contains intravenous catheters, different solutions, and different administration settings.

Medication: Both for advanced life support and basic life support, paramedics carry a wide variety of drugs in their kits. It is essential to have knowledge of the indications, dosages, and side effects associated with various medications.

equipment for Splinting and Immobilization Paramedics employ equipment such as backboards, cervical collars, and splints on patients who have fractures or spinal injuries in order to immobilize and stabilize the patients.

3. Automobiles:

The following categories of motor vehicles are among those that paramedic services use:

Ambulances come in two different types: type I, which is built on a truck chassis and includes a roomy interior for patient care, and type III, which is smaller and built on a van chassis. Ambulances of the Type III variety are constructed on van chassis and have a more compact design. Both varieties provide unique benefits that are well-suited to a variety of clinical settingss and patient demographics.

Units Specializing in Critical Care, newborn Care, or Bariatric Patients Some emergency medical services have specialist units for the evacuation of patients requiring critical care, newborn care, or bariatric care.

All-Terrain Vehicles (ATVs) and Bicycle Units: In certain circumstances, paramedics may use ATVs or bicycles to reach patients in surroundings that are difficult to navigate or that are crowded.

Systematization of Communication and Information

In order for paramedic operations to be successful, effective communication and information management are essential components. In order to coordinate care, disseminate information about patients, and document their actions, paramedics rely on a variety of systems, including the following:

1. Electronic Patient Care Records, abbreviated as "ePCRs"

Traditional paper-based patient records have been replaced with electronic patient care records (ePCRs), which enable paramedics to electronically enter patient data, vital signs, and actions. ePCRs make it easier to share data with hospitals and other healthcare professionals, which speeds up the treatment process for patients.

2. Communications in the Hospital:

Communicating with the hospitals that are receiving patients allows for the provision of patient information, the request of consultations, and the receipt of orders. For a smooth handoff of patients, it is necessary to maintain effective communication with the staff of the emergency department.

3. Capability of Interoperability:

Interoperability is the capacity of separate computer systems to collaborate and exchange information with one another. It is the goal of paramedic services to achieve interoperability between their electronic patient care record (ePCR) systems, radio communications, and hospital information systems in order to facilitate the effective transmission of patient data.

Initiatives for the Improvement of Quality

The provision of patient care and the effectiveness of paramedic services is continuously the focus of research and development efforts. Initiatives for quality improvement include monitoring, reviewing, and improving many different elements of paramedic services, including the following:

1. Supervision by the Medical Director:

The operation of paramedic services is directed by a medical director, who is responsible for providing clinical oversight, developing guidelines, and ensuring that evidence-based practices are adhered to at all times. The medical director is responsible for playing an important part in the process of quality improvement.

2. Ongoing Training and Education:

Education and training for paramedics is continuous, as it is necessary for them to be up to date on the most recent advancements that have been made in clinical practice, equipment, and protocols. Continuing education is absolutely necessary in order to keep the high standards of care that have been established.

3. Metrics Regarding Performance:

Performance metrics are devised by paramedic services in order to evaluate many facets of their operations, such as the length of response times, the clinical outcomes, and the level of patient satisfaction. Monitoring these parameters enables data-driven improvements, which can then be implemented.

4. Audits and Reviews of Clinical Practice:

Clinical audits and reviews are carried out on a consistent basis in order to assess individual cases and locate areas in which there is room for advancement. The resuscitation of cardiac arrest victims, the treatment of stroke victims, or any number of other life-saving procedures could be the subject of these audits.

5. Research and New Product Development:

In order to investigate new treatment modalities and the most effective methods in the field of paramedicine, paramedic services may take part in research projects and work in collaboration with academic institutions.

Participation in the Community

Education and participation in the community are extremely important responsibilities that fall to paramedic services. These activities include of things like:

1. Education in the Public Sector:

Community members, schools, and companies can benefit from the education that paramedics offer on a variety of topics, including cardiopulmonary resuscitation (CPR), first aid, injury prevention, and disaster preparedness.

2. Community-Based Programs in the Field of Paramedicine:

The scope of services provided by paramedics is broadened through the implementation of community paramedicine initiatives. The provision of preventative care, the management of chronic diseases, and post-discharge follow-up in the community are the primary focuses of these initiatives.

3. Preparation for Catastrophes:

The development of disaster response plans and the preparation of emergency management agencies to respond to large-scale emergencies and natural disasters is a collaborative effort between paramedics and emergency management authorities.

4. Efforts to Improve Public Safety:

Participation in public safety initiatives that raise awareness and encourage safe behaviors—for example, the use of seatbelts and helmets, as well as the perils of driving while impaired—may be open to paramedic services.

Exercise Tests are covered in Chapter 12.

If you want to become a paramedic, taking practice exams is an essential part of the process. Not only do they help you get ready for the National Registry Paramedic (NRP) certification, but they also ensure that you have the information and abilities required to offer high-quality pre-hospital care. This chapter will give you with sample practice questions to help you test your knowledge and build confidence in your abilities, as well as take you through the significance of practice tests, how to make effective use of them, and how to use them efficiently.

The Value of Taking Several Practice Tests

The education of paramedics and the preparation for their certification both heavily rely on the taking of practice examinations. They provide a number of benefits that will add to your success, including the following:

Evaluation of Knowledge Taking practice exams allows you to evaluate how well you grasp the topic and identifies areas in which you can benefit from additional study.

Exposure to the Format of the Exam Being familiar with the format and structure of the NRP certification exam will help lessen test anxiety and increase your ability to perform well on tests.

Time Management: Taking practice tests will help you learn how to manage your time during the real exam, which will ensure that you have sufficient time to answer all of the questions.

Application of Knowledge You'll need to demonstrate that you can apply what you've learned in the classroom to real-world situations in order to pass the practice examinations. These situations should be similar to those that you'll encounter in the field.

Building Confidence Doing Well on Practice examinations Can Boost Your Self-Confidence and Reduce Test-Related Stress Doing well on practice examinations can make you feel more confident going into the real thing.

Identifying Weaknesses Doing a self-assessment by analyzing your performance on practice examinations will help you identify areas in which you may require further study and review.

Review and Reinforcement: Going through practice questions gives you the opportunity to review and reinforce the information you've learned as well as make any required adjustments to your study strategy.

How to Make the Most Out of Your Practice Exams

Consider the following tactics when taking practice tests so that you may get the most out of them:

Create a Routine for Your Studies: Prepare for mock examinations in the same manner as you would for real study sessions by blocking off particular hours for them. The key to successful preparing for the exam is consistency.

In order to simulate the conditions of the real exam, you should conduct your practice tests in an area that is free from any potential distractions. Prepare yourself for the time limits of the real exam by setting a timer.

Make Use of Official Resources You should look for official practice tests and study materials that are offered by the National Registry of Emergency Medical Technicians (NREMT). These are geared at the actual NRP examination that you will take.

Pay Attention to Weak Areas: After you have completed a practice test, go back and look through the questions that you got wrong. Focus on the subject areas in which you had the most trouble and look for additional study resources to help you with those topics.

Change the Sources of Your Questions You should take your practice examinations from a variety of sources including traditional textbooks, online question banks, and study aids. This offers a more comprehensive view of the various questions that could appear on the exam.

Keep a Log: Make sure to keep a log of your scores on your practice exams and make a note of any improvements. Monitoring your advancement can be an effective way to motivate yourself and can also assist you in determining which aspects of your performance still require improvement.

Rationales for Review The majority of the time, the practice tests that you take will include explanations or rationales for the right answers. Read through these justifications to have an understanding of why certain answers are correct.

You should schedule a day specifically for taking a full-length practice exam, during which you should try to replicate the conditions of the actual examination as nearly as you can. This prepares you to feel more comfortable with the format of the exam.

Request Feedback: If it is at all possible, seek a paramedic instructor or mentor to review the outcomes of your practice exams and provide feedback on the areas of your performance that need to be improved.

Examples of Questions to Be Used in Practice

Let's have a look at some examples of practice questions that address the important concepts that you've been learning about throughout this book. First, you should evaluate your level of comprehension by working through the questions, and then you should look over the explanations.

Please take into consideration that these questions are intended solely for the purpose of practice and do not in any way reflect the actual content of the NRP certification exam. It is absolutely necessary to reference official NRP study resources and practice examinations in order to get the best possible representation of the subject that will be on the exam.

1. Evaluation of the Patient

You are dispatched to the scene of a call about a man in his forties who is complaining of chest trouble. During the primary assessment, you notice that the patient is aware, but that they are in a great deal of pain. His skin is clammy and sweaty at the same time. He is having trouble breathing and is complaining of pain in the chest. Which component of the assessment should you give the most weight to?

B. Ensure that a carotid pulse is present.

A. Give high-flow oxygen to the patient.

C. Perform a thorough assessment of the patient's airway, breathing, and circulation.

D. Obtain a complete medical history of the patient.

The correct answer is option C, which is to evaluate the patient's airway, breathing, and circulation.

When a patient comes in complaining of chest discomfort and distress, the most important thing to do is to evaluate the patient's airway, breathing, and circulation (also known as the ABCs) in order to diagnose and treat any potentially life-threatening disorders. It's possible that giving the patient oxygen and getting a complete medical history will come next, but the most important thing is to make sure they survive the immediate crisis.

2. The study of pharmaceuticals

You are providing medical care for a patient who is undergoing a very severe allergic reaction. What kind of drug is used as the initial line of defense against anaphylaxis?

A. Albuterol, also known as Ventolin

Epinephrine, component B

Benadryl, also known as C. Diphenhydramine

Nitroglycerin, the letter D

The correct answer is epinephrine (B).

Since epinephrine may swiftly reverse the severe symptoms of an allergic reaction, it is the therapy of choice for anaphylaxis, the most severe form of a severe allergic reaction. The bronchodilator albuterol, the antihistamine diphenhydramine, and the chest pain medication nitroglycerin are the three most common uses for these three medications.

3. Clinical Cardiology

A woman in her sixties reports to the emergency room complaining of excruciating chest discomfort that is radiating to her left arm and is accompanied by profuse sweating. Her pulse is 110 beats per minute, and her respirations are happening at a rate of 20 per minute. Her blood pressure is 180 over 100 mm Hg. What is the most likely diagnosis, and how should one first go about treating this condition?

Myocardial infarction is present; aspirin and nitroglycerin should be given. A.

Aortic dissection; nitroglycerin should be given, and pain medication should be administered.

C. Congestive heart failure; furosemide and oxygen therapy should be administered.

D. Attack of anxiety; provide diazepam to the patient.

Myocardial infarction is the correct diagnosis; aspirin and nitroglycerin should be given.

Explanation: The symptoms that the patient is exhibiting strongly point to the presence of a myocardial infarction (also known as a heart attack). Aspirin, which inhibits platelet aggregation, and nitroglycerin, which provides relief from chest pain, should be part of the initial treatment. These precautions assist reduce the severity of the damage done to the heart.

4. Shock and Awe

The fourth scenario has you arriving at the site of a motorcycle accident. The rider, a male who is 25 years old, is conscious but in a great deal of agony. It seems as though he has shattered and disfigured his left leg. There are no further injuries that pose a threat to his life. Which of the following would be the best first step to take with this patient?

A. Give the patient the appropriate medication to alleviate the pain.

B. Apply a splint or a SAM splint to the left leg in order to keep it from moving.

C. Put a tourniquet on the wound to stop the bleeding.

D. Start chest compressions and defibrillation.

Answer: B. Apply a splint or a SAM splint to the left leg in order to keep it from moving.

The application of a splint on the patient's left leg in order to keep the leg from moving and reduce the patient's level of discomfort should be the patient's first priority. After the patient has been immobilized, pain medication should be given; this should not be the first thing that is done. Because there is not a significant risk of life-threatening bleeding, a tourniquet is not necessary for this patient. It is not necessary to do cardiopulmonary resuscitation (CPR) or defibrillation on a trauma patient who is conscious.

5. The specialties of Obstetrics and Pediatrics

You have been dispatched to assist a pregnant woman of 32 years of age who is currently going through active labor. She lets you know that this is her first pregnancy and that she is having contractions every 5 minutes. Additionally, she says that she is feeling quite uncomfortable. Upon closer inspection, you notice that she has reached her complete dilation and is now ready to give birth. What steps should you take after this?

A. Take steps to make the patient more comfortable and convince her that you will take her to the hospital as soon as possible.

B. Contribute to the procedure of the delivery.

C. Administer medication to alleviate the pain.

D. Apply a tocolytic drug in order to postpone the labor process.

Answer: B. Contribute to the procedure of delivering the goods.

When a pregnant patient is fully dilated and ready to give birth, you should assist with the delivery process so that the birth goes as smoothly as possible. In this particular circumstance, it is essential to provide both passive and active aid in addition to comfort measures and reassurance. During the second stage of labor, pain relieving medicine is not given, and instead tocolytic medications are utilized to delay labor, which is not appropriate in this circumstance.

Review of the Entire Chapter and Strategies for the Day of the Exam

It is crucial to consolidate your knowledge, review key ideas, and prepare yourself both mentally and physically for the National Registry Paramedic (NRP) certification exam as you get closer to the end of your education and training as a paramedic. This chapter will walk you through the final review process and provide crucial test-day ideas to help you achieve your goal of becoming a certified paramedic.

Complete Examination

Your readiness for the NRP certification exam will benefit greatly from the comprehensive review you have just completed. It gives you the opportunity to review and improve the knowledge and abilities you've gained throughout the course of your study to become a paramedic. The following is an in-depth walkthrough of how to successfully complete the final review:

Determine the Most Important Subject Areas and Topics First, you should determine the most important subject areas and topics that are likely to be covered on the NRP exam. Assessment of patients, pharmacology, cardiology, trauma, obstetrics, pediatrics, and surgical procedures are some examples of these specialties. Conduct a thorough examination of your reading materials and the subject matter covered in the course.

Make a Timetable for Your Studies: Create a study program for the final review session, which will often encompass several weeks leading up to the exam. This period will be right before the test. Time should be set out specifically for each subject area, and this should be determined by your initial assessment of where your strengths and limitations lie.

Use the Official Study Materials You should rely on the official study materials and practice exams provided by the NRP. These resources have been meticulously crafted to correspond with the structure and content of the NRP examination. They provide the most accurate portrayal of what you might expect to see on the actual examination.

Exams for Practice It is recommended that you complete practice exams sourced from official sources as well as other credible vendors. Make use of these exams to evaluate your knowledge, determine areas in which you could improve, and get a feel for the structure of the examination.

Pay Extra Attention to Weak Areas: Devote more of your time and energy to the subject areas in which you performed less well on sample tests or in which you have less self-assurance. To further your comprehension, go back over the relevant textbooks, reference books, and other reading material.

Concepts Crucial to Understand It is important to review certain essential ideas, methods, and treatment protocols. You should make sure that you have a solid understanding of the reasoning behind each operation or intervention before taking the exam, as this will help you with both multiple-choice questions and scenario-based questions.

Participate in Active Learning: If you want to learn more effectively, you should participate in active learning rather than simply reading or viewing study materials. Constructing flashcards, giving yourself quizzes, and taking part in group study sessions are all excellent ways to solidify your grasp of the material.

Clinical Scenarios: To gain experience in dealing with real-life scenarios that paramedics really encounter, students work through clinical scenarios. Applying what you've learned and improving your ability to think critically will both benefit you from doing this.

Time Management: Be sure to keep a close eye on your time management during the practice exams. Because you will need to demonstrate this ability on the real NRP exam, you should make sure that you finish each section within the allocated time.

Maintain Current Knowledge: It is important to be informed of any current modifications or changes that have been made to the protocols, equipment, or medications used in paramedic care. Make sure that your learning materials reflect the most recent recommendations.

Seek Direction: If you have access to paramedic instructors or mentors, consult with them to seek direction and clarification on any difficult subjects that you may be struggling with.

Strategies for the Day of the Exam

The day of the test can be nerve-wracking, but if you prepare yourself properly, you can maximize both your performance and your confidence. Think about using these tactics on the day of the test:

go There Early: Make it a priority to go to the testing center in plenty of time before the start of your examination. This will give you time to check in, complete any documentation that is necessary, and mentally prepare yourself for what is to come.

Valid Identification and authorisation: Ensure that you have a valid picture identification card issued by the government as well as any necessary authorisation paperwork. If you do not bring these items, you risk being denied access to the exam.

Bring Necessary Items Prepare a compact bag or case with necessary items such as identity, authorization, a watch, pencils or pens, and a silent, non-programmable, non-photographic calculator (if authorized) and bring these things with you.

Dress Comfy: Because you may not be able to manage the temperature of the room, you should dress in layers so that you are comfortable. Layering up your clothing gives you the ability to adapt to a variety of climates.

Keep Yourself Hydrated and Nourished Before the test, eat a meal that is light but well-balanced, and drink plenty of water to keep yourself hydrated. It is important to steer clear of foods and beverages that are dense, high in sugar, or include caffeine because these can cause energy dumps throughout the exam.

Get a full night's sleep the night before the test to make sure that you are both mentally and physically refreshed when you show up. If you discover that you are experiencing anxiety, try practicing some relaxation techniques such as meditation or deep breathing.

Observe the directions: Both before and while you are taking the exam, pay very close attention to the directions that are provided by the employees at the testing center. They will offer direction regarding the procedure for the test, as well as any unique rules.

Time management is essential, as there is a strict limit on how long you have to complete the NRP exam. It is important to go quickly through the questions and to avoid becoming stuck on difficult issues. Mark any questions that you are unable to answer and come back to them later if you have time.

Take Your Time to Read: Carefully read each question and the available response choices. Pay close attention to the question itself, particularly the phrases and specifics that could help direct your response.

Elimination Method: If you are unsure about an answer, you can use the elimination method to eliminate possibilities that are blatantly incorrect. Your chances of selecting the appropriate solution may improve as a result of doing so.

Strategic Guessing If you come across a question that you don't know the answer to, you should make an educated guess based on the information you know and the context of the question. Guessing is not punished in the vast majority of examinations.

Mark and Review: If the software for the exam permits you to, mark questions that you are unclear about so that you can review them later. After you have finished the first time through the test, you should go back through the questions that were marked and rethink your responses.

During the test, it is important to have a level head and keep your concentration. Pacing yourself and concentrating on answering one question at a time will help you avoid feeling unduly stressed.

Questions Based on Scenarios: When answering questions based on scenarios, you should approach them as if you were in the field. Think through the procedures you would follow if you were providing care for a real patient.

Multiple-Choice Questions: When answering multiple-choice questions, first remove the answers that are patently incorrect, and then select the most appropriate response from among the alternatives that are left.

Be mindful of the Time, and Pace Yourself Appropriately Be mindful of the time, and pace yourself appropriately. You shouldn't spend an excessive amount of time on any one question or section. Make finishing all of the sections your first priority.

Maintain a Positive Attitude: Always try to see the bright side of things and have faith in your skills and knowledge. Having a constructive outlook on the test can make it easier for you to complete it.

Before you hand in your test, you should go back over your answers and make sure that you've covered everything by checking all the appropriate boxes. Check to see that you haven't overlooked any of the items by accident.

Don't Waste Time Guessing: After you've handed in your test, don't waste time thinking about the questions. The past can't be changed, and there's no point in second-guessing the decisions you've already made.

After the Exam Thoughts and Questions

After passing the NRP certification exam, there are a few things to think about in the post-exam period, including the following:

Be Prepared to Wait for Your Results: There will be a Waiting Period Before Your Exam Results Are Released to You. In most cases, the results of the NRP can be obtained within a few days to a few weeks.

Continuing Education: Regardless of whether you pass or fail the exam, you should strongly consider participating in continuing education in order to keep up with the most recent breakthroughs in the field of paramedicine. To keep your certification current, you are required to complete continuing education units.

Review Weak Areas: If you do not succeed in passing the test, you should concentrate on the areas in which you performed the worst and then participate in focused study and practice in those areas. After a certain amount of time has passed, you will be able to repeat the exam.

Take Some Time to Celebrate Your Success If you are successful in passing the exam and obtaining your paramedic certification, you should take some time to congratulate yourself on your accomplishment. This is an important turning point in your professional journey.

Resources and supplementary learning aids are covered in Chapter 14.

If you want to become a paramedic, having access to high-quality resources and learning aids can make a big difference in how well you learn and how well you prepare for the National Registry of Paramedics (NRP) certification exam. This chapter will present a comprehensive list of resources, both online and in print, to assist you in furthering your education as a paramedic and improving your chances of successfully achieving your certification.

The Best Online Sources

Website of the National Registry of Emergency Medical Technicians (NREMT): The official website is the major source for information on NRP certification, including exam instructions, registration information, and study tools. You may find this information on the NREMT website. Website of the NREMT

Sheets for the NREMT Psychomotor Exam for Paramedics: You should review the practical skills that will be examined on the NRP exam by accessing the official psychomotor exam papers. Sheets for the Psychomotor Exam

Exam to Practice for the NREMT Paramedic Certification The NREMT provides a sample exam to help candidates become accustomed to the structure and content of the certification examination. Practice Exam for the Paramedic Position

NREMT Handbook: The official NREMT handbook is a helpful resource that offers thorough information on the NRP certification process, exam content, and requirements. This book can be found on the NREMT website. Manual of the NREMT

EMS1 is a website that provides a multitude of articles, videos, and other materials that are associated with emergency medical services (EMS) and paramedicine. EMS1

JEMS stands for the "Journal of Emergency Medical Services," and it is a publication that offers a variety of papers, case studies, and clinical information that is connected to pre-hospital care and paramedicine. JEMS

EMS World: EMS World is yet another online resource for emergency medical services workers, providing them with news, articles, webinars, and other forms of instructional content. A World of EMS

EMT-Paramedic.com: EMT-Paramedic.com is a website that provides a variety of study resources for paramedics, such as practice examinations, flashcards, and study guides. The EMT-Paramedic.com website.

The phrase "paramedic tutor" refers to a company that offers online courses and study materials to paramedic students who are getting ready for their certification examinations. Instructor of Paramedics

The Prehospital Care Research Forum (PCRF) is an organization that provides a collection of research and resources that are associated with emergency medical services (EMS). PCRF

UpToDate is a clinical decision support resource that is utilized all around the world by various types of medical practitioners. It is able to offer comprehensive information on a variety of medical topics as well as treatment suggestions. There may be a subscription fee required to gain access. Current and ongoing

Textbooks and Other Printed Materials

"Paramedic Care: Principles & Practice" Lecture Series: This collection of textbooks on paramedicine covers everything from anatomy and physiology to patient assessment and trauma, as well as a variety of other topics, and was written by Bryan E. Bledsoe and other recognized authorities.

"Nancy Caroline's Emergency Care in the Streets" is a thorough textbook that is an essential component of paramedic education. It covers a wide variety of subjects that are pertinent to pre-hospital care and is an industry standard.

"Emergency Medical Responder: First on Scene" : Even though it was written specifically for Emergency Medical Responders (EMRs), this textbook can be an extremely helpful resource for paramedic students who are looking to reaffirm their knowledge of fundamental concepts.

Textbooks for Paramedics Offered by "Brady Books" Brady Books is home to a wide selection of paramedic textbooks, some of which include "Paramedic Emergency Care" and "Paramedic Practice Today."

This literature, which is known by its acronym PHTLS and stands for "Prehospital Trauma Life Support," offers in-depth information on the evaluation and treatment of trauma, which is an essential part of paramedic work.

"ACLS Provider Manual": The Advanced Cardiovascular Life Support (ACLS) provider manual is crucial for paramedics, as ACLS is an essential skill in emergency care.

"PALS Provider Manual": The Pediatric Advanced Life Support (PALS) provider manual is an essential resource for paramedics who may be called upon to treat pediatric patients in the event of an emergency.

"Neonatal Resuscitation Program": If you plan to offer care to neonates, the manual for the Neonatal Resuscitation Program is absolutely necessary to read in order to gain an awareness of the specific requirements that apply to infants.

Applications as well as Mobile Resources

EMT Tutor Lite is a smartphone app that provides students studying to become EMTs or paramedics with practice questions and flashcards. It is downloadable for use on both iOS and Android devices.

EMT PASS: EMT PASS is an app that helps emergency medical technicians and paramedics prepare for their certification exams by giving both practice questions and in-depth explanations of the correct answers.

ACLS Fast-Track: This program was developed specifically for the purpose of preparing users for the ACLS certification exam by providing practice algorithms and scenarios.

PALS Advisor is a mobile app that provides pediatric resuscitation guidelines, algorithms, and quick references. PALS Advisor was created by the Pediatric Advanced Life Support (PALS) program.

Calculate by QxMD is a helpful medical calculator program that provides assistance with medicine dosages, clinical tools, and medical equations.

Provider of Paramedic Protocols: This application provides paramedic protocols for a variety of places and assists you in keeping up to speed with the most recent set of local standards.

Anki: Anki is a digital flashcard program that enables users to design and review their own flashcards, making it a versatile learning tool for students studying to become paramedics.

YouTube: Although it is not an app, YouTube contains a large number of educational channels and videos on a variety of themes related to paramedicine, including demonstrations of various procedures and explanations of difficult concepts.

Discussion Groups and Online Forums

Join the NREMT Study Group on Facebook to make connections with other students studying to become paramedics, discuss study strategies, and exchange information about available resources. Study Group for the NREMT

The EMS Student subreddit is a place for students and professionals to discuss subjects relating to emergency medical services (EMS) education and paramedicine. EMS Student Community on Reddit

EMT City is an online community that brings together EMS professionals and students to discuss a variety of subjects that are all connected to the field of emergency medical services. The EMT City

JEMS Connect is a community forum hosted by the Journal of Emergency Medical Services (JEMS) that brings together EMS professionals for the purpose of networking and discussing issues that are pertinent to the industry. JEMS Connect (JEMS)

Additional Instructions and Methods for Studying

Active Learning: Instead of passively absorbing information, actively engage in the process of learning by doing things like making flashcards, testing oneself, and teaching the content to others.

Study Groups Students in the paramedic program are encouraged to form or join existing study groups. Your comprehension can improve through participation in group discussions and the instruction of others.

Real-World Scenarios: Putting your knowledge to use requires practice with real-world scenarios. Particularly beneficial might be the use of simulation exercises.

In order to effectively manage your time, devise a study plan that allots predetermined amounts of time to various themes or fields of inquiry. This enables you to effectively cover all of the content.

Mnemonics and Acronyms: To remember difficult algorithms, drug dosages, and evaluation processes, use mnemonics and acronyms.

Exam Preparation: You should try to complete as many practice examinations as you can. They will familiarize you with the format of the exam and test your knowledge of the material.

Maintain a Current Knowledge Base: Always check for new paramedicine guidelines and information as it becomes available. It is essential to be educated because medical protocols are subject to change.

Maintaining a Healthy Lifestyle: In order to maintain a healthy lifestyle, it is important to eat a balanced diet, regularly engage in physical activity, and get enough sleep. greater cognitive performance is associated with greater physical health.

Mental Preparation: Give your mind a workout in preparation for the test. Anxiety can be alleviated via the use of relaxation techniques and by having positive self-talk.

Ask for Help: If there is a particular issue that you are having trouble understanding, do not be afraid to ask for assistance from your paramedic professors, mentors, or classmates.

Special Populations is the focus of Chapter 15.

The training that paramedics get prepares them to give emergency medical assistance to a wide variety of patients, including members of special populations who have specific medical requirements. This chapter examines the issues, problems, and best practices for providing care to unique populations. These populations include pregnant patients, pediatric patients, geriatric patients, and individuals with disabilities. Other special populations include pregnant patients and individuals with disabilities.

Patients of Childhood Age

Providing medical attention to pediatric patients calls for a one-of-a-kind strategy due to the fact that children and adults display physiological, psychological, and developmental distinctions that are distinct from one another. The following are important things to keep in mind when treating pediatric patients:

Assessment and Communication: When communicating with children, use language that is appropriate for their age and present a manner that is calm and soothing. Conduct a thorough examination of the youngsters, paying particular attention to any indicators of distress, particularly difficulty breathing and circulation.

Medication Administration Based on Weight: When giving medication to a child, it is best to base the dosage either on the child's weight or on the child's body surface area. Be knowledgeable about the appropriate dosing and computations for pediatric patients.

Management of Pain: In the event of a medical emergency, children frequently experience both pain and worry. Make sure you use pain assessment scales that are age-appropriate for the patient, and give them pain treatment as needed.

When dealing with a child, it is important to take into account where the child is in his or her development. There are distinct differences in the types of requirements and modes of communication that are required by infants, toddlers, school-aged children, and teenagers.

Involvement of the Family: In order to acquire the child's medical history and to offer emotional support, it is important to involve the child's parents or guardians. It is important to keep the family updated on the child's condition and treatment at all times.

Equipment Specifically Designed for Children Ensure that your ambulance is stocked with equipment designed specifically for children, such as smaller blood pressure cuffs, pediatric defibrillator pads, and appropriate airway devices.

Neonatal Resuscitation: If you are called to a delivery or a neonatal emergency, you should always be prepared to do neonatal resuscitation. It is absolutely necessary to be familiar with the Neonatal Resuscitation Program (NRP).

Abuse and Neglect of Children: It is important to remain watchful for any indicators of child abuse or neglect. It is absolutely necessary to preserve the health and safety of children to report any suspicious or concerning behavior to the paramedics who respond to the scene.

Patients of an Elderly Age

Providing medical attention to elderly patients presents a distinct set of issues due to the fact that older people are more likely to have several chronic conditions and specific requirements:

Polypharmacy is the practice in which geriatric adults take many drugs at once. Examine their medication history and ask them questions about it because drug interactions and side effects might result in serious medical problems.

Falls: Older persons have a higher risk of falling, which can lead to broken bones, brain injuries, or internal bleeding. Falls can sometimes be fatal. Be sure to do an exhaustive assessment, and if necessary, think about taking spinal precautions.

When working with patients who have dementia or cognitive impairment, it is important to exhibit patience and empathy for their situation. Make sure they are safe and respect their dignity at all times.

Diseases that last a long time Many older patients suffer from conditions that last a long time, such as diabetes, hypertension, or heart disease. Recognize the indicators of decompensation and ensure that the patient receives the necessary care.

Do not forget to educate yourself about do-not-resuscitate (DNR) orders and advance directives. Respect the patient's desires at all times while remaining compliant with all applicable laws and ethical standards.

Functional Decline It is important to evaluate the patient's current functional state as well as their mobility. Address any issues with movement and provide additional support, such as steps to prevent falls.

Pain Management It's possible that elderly folks will suffer from persistent pain. It is essential for their comfort and overall wellbeing to have adequate pain management.

End-of-Life Care: When it becomes clear that the patient is nearing the end of their life, compassionate end-of-life care should be provided. Palliative care should also be considered, and the patient's emotional and psychological needs should be met.

Patients who have various impairments

It is imperative that paramedics be trained to provide medical assistance to people with a variety of impairments, including those that are intellectual, sensory, physical, and developmental in nature:

Communication: Adjust your mode of communication so that it takes into account the unique limitation that the patient has. Make use of sign language, for instance, when dealing with patients who have hearing difficulties, and pictorial communication when dealing with non-verbal individuals.

Mobility: Be ready to assist with mobility aids such as wheelchairs or walkers, and offer appropriate fastening inside the ambulance for these items. When necessary, make sure there are accessible options for getting around.

Impairments to the Senses Patients who have impairments to their senses may require the use of assistive technologies or service animals. It is imperative that you look out for the health and safety of these patients, including their service animals.

Problems with Behavior It's possible that some people who have intellectual or developmental difficulties will also have problems with their behavior. In order to bring the level of tension in a scenario down, it is important to remain cool and avoid confrontation.

administration of Medications: Patients who have disabilities may need support with the administration of their medications. Check the patient's medication schedule and look for any potential drug interactions.

Cultural Competence It is important to have cultural competence and to be aware of the specific requirements of people with disabilities who come from a variety of cultural backgrounds.

Legal Protections: Become familiar with the Americans with Disabilities Act (ADA) and its provisions for accessible facilities and services. This act was passed in 1990.

Patients Who Are Pregnant

To be able to provide treatment to pregnant patients, one must have a grasp of the physiological shifts that occur throughout pregnancy as well as the potential difficulties that can occur during childbirth:

Find out how far along you are in your pregnancy by calculating your gestational age. This information is essential for determining the appropriate course of action and any potential difficulties.

Positioning: When pregnant patients are being examined, it is best to have them lie on their left side so that more blood can reach the fetus. Steer clear of supine positions since they can cause the vena cava to become compressed.

Be on the lookout for indicators of preterm labor, like as contractions, bleeding in the uterine lining, and ruptured membranes, and make sure you get enough of rest. It is critical to quickly recognize the condition and take the patient to the right clinic.

Check for eclampsia, a potentially fatal illness characterized by seizures in pregnant women. eclampsia can cause miscarriage or stillbirth. Recognize the symptoms, such as extreme hypertension and seizures, and begin emergency treatment as soon as possible.

Assistance with Delivery Paramedics may be called upon to provide delivery assistance in certain situations. Maintain compliance with the predetermined procedures, and offer the mother your support throughout the labor and delivery process.

Monitoring of the Fetal Heart Rate During prehospital treatment, it is important to use a fetal heart rate monitor in order to determine whether or not the fetus is doing okay. Urgent action is required as soon as the fetal heart rate drops below the normal range or disappears entirely.

Patient Position: In the event that the patient is about to give birth, you should position them for delivery and provide support, such as helping the infant with their head.

Preparation for newborn Care It is important to be ready for newborn care, which includes the management of airways and neonatal resuscitation. The health of the baby can be evaluated with the use of the Apgar score.

Competence and sensitivity across cultural contexts

In any circumstance, it is absolutely necessary to address specific groups of people with cultural competence and sensitivity. It is important to be respectful of the patient's personal, cultural, and religious beliefs. The following are components of cultural competence:

Effective communication involves communicating in a way that is both clear and respectful, taking into account any language obstacles that may exist as well as the patient's chosen method of communication.

Understanding culture Beliefs and Practices It is important to have an understanding of the culture beliefs, practices, and healthcare expectations. Some societies, for instance, can have particular preferences for herbal medicines or traditional healers.

Involvement of Families and Communities: Many different cultures place a high value on the participation of family or community members in the decision-making process about medical care. Pay respect to these people and include them when it's suitable.

Modesty and Privacy: When working with patients from cultures that place a high importance on modesty and privacy, it is important to maintain sensitivity to these issues.

Religious Accommodations: Whenever it is possible, try to accommodate the patients' various religious practices, such as food restrictions or the requirements of prayer.

A patient's advance directives and preferences should be respected, and it should be ensured that their values and beliefs are respected while they are receiving care.

Avoiding Stereotyping It is important to refrain from generalizing about patients' ethnic or demographic backgrounds and to avoid forming assumptions about them. Always consider the patient to be an individual.

Emergencies Related to the Environment, Section 16

Environmental emergencies are a general term referring to a variety of medical conditions that are either brought on by the environment or made worse by it. Patients who are facing various environmental emergencies, which can range from illnesses caused by heat exposure to illnesses caused by cold exposure, as well as drowning, and more, are regularly seen by paramedics. This chapter discusses the environmental emergencies that are most likely to be encountered by paramedics, as well as the best ways to evaluate and deal with these situations.

Illnesses Associated with Heat

When the body's ability to control its temperature is overpowered by variables from the environment, most frequently high levels of heat and humidity, heat-related disorders can develop. The severity of these diseases can range from relatively harmless heat cramps to potentially fatal heat stroke. Among the most common heat-related ailments are:

Heat Cramps: Heat cramps are painful muscle contractions that often arise from engaging in strenuous physical activity while the temperature is high. The treatment consists of repositioning the patient in a cooler environment, giving them fluids, and gently stretching them.

Heat exhaustion is characterized by profuse perspiration, weakness, dizziness, nausea, and a rapid heartbeat. Other symptoms of heat exhaustion include heat stroke. The patient needs to be removed from the heat, they need to have their fluids replaced, and the condition of the patient needs to be monitored.

A medical emergency known as heat stroke takes place when the internal temperature of the body increases to an unsafely high level. Heat stroke can be fatal. Confusion, fast breathing, and a lack of sweating are all signs and symptoms of this condition. It is imperative that paramedics quickly administer supportive treatment and cool the patient.

Emergencies Connected to the Cold

Emergencies caused by exposure to cold temperatures can lead to a variety of conditions, including frostbite and hypothermia, as well as other potentially life-threatening outcomes:

Frostbite is a condition that happens when the tissues of the body freeze, resulting in harm to those tissues. Patients could feel tingling, numbness, or pain in the areas that are affected by the condition. The patient needs to be rapidly rewarmed, but this process must be carried out with extreme caution in order to avoid further injury.

Hypothermia is a potentially fatal condition that occurs when the body loses heat at a rate that is greater than the rate at which it can produce heat. Shaking, bewilderment, and a sluggish heart rate are all symptoms of this condition. If the patient is aware, emergency medical technicians should gradually rewarm them, handle them carefully, and give them warm fluids.

Almost drowning and then actually drowning

Around the world, drowning is a leading cause of accidental death and permanent disability. The term "near drowning" refers to a situation in which a person comes dangerously close to drowning but manages to live. When dealing with cases of drowning, the following are important considerations:

Perform a rescue that is both quick and secure, then evaluate the situation. After the patient has been removed from the water, an assessment of their respiration and circulation should be performed. It is possible that the patient need immediate cardiopulmonary resuscitation (CPR).

Aspiration Pneumonia: When people drown, they frequently breathe water into their lungs, which can cause aspiration pneumonia. Keep an eye out for any signs of respiratory distress and administer treatment as needed.

Time Spent Underwater The length of time a person is under water is a significant factor in determining their prognosis. It has been found that longer periods of submersion are related with poorer outcomes.

Hypothermia is a condition that can rapidly develop when exposed to water, particularly cold water. Carefully rewarm the patient, offering warm fluids as needed, and provide close attention to the patient.

Secondary Drowning: Even after a patient has made an initial recovery from drowning, there is still a chance that they will develop delayed problems. Always be on the lookout for secondary symptoms of drowning, such as coughing, chest pain, and difficulty breathing.

There was a lightning strike.

There is a wide range of injuries that can be caused by lightning strikes, ranging from mild burns to cardiac arrest. When assisting those who have been struck by lightning, you should:

Before approaching the patient, make sure the situation has been cleared of any potential dangers, such as future lightning strikes.

Lightning has been shown to interfere with the normal electrical activity of the heart, which can result in cardiac arrest. Perform cardiopulmonary resuscitation (CPR), and if necessary, use an automated external defibrillator (AED).

Burns can occur as a result of lightning, both at the point of entry and the point of escape. Carefully evaluate the burns and treat them in accordance with their severity.

Neurological Effects: There is a possibility that some individuals will develop neurological effects, such as confusion, a loss of memory, or even post-concussion syndrome. Ensure that a complete neurological assessment is performed.

Shock: People who are struck by lightning may fall into shock, which requires immediate medical attention in order to keep their circulation and blood pressure stable.

The Bites and Stings of Animals and Insects

Bites and stings by animals and insects can result in a variety of adverse health effects, including allergic reactions and infections:

Anaphylaxis is a severe allergic reaction that can be triggered by some bites and stings from insects and animals. Epinephrine should be given, and prompt advanced treatment should be provided for those who are experiencing anaphylaxis.

Infection: Bites, particularly those from mammals, have the potential to transfer germs into the wound, which can then lead to infection. Make sure the wound is clean and apply the appropriate dressing.

Rabies is a disease that can be transmitted through animal bites, most commonly those received from wild animals. Investigate the identity of the animal that bit you, as post-exposure prophylaxis can be required in some cases.

Toxic effects of plants

Poisoning from plants can occur either through consumption of the plants or through contact with them. It is vital to be familiar with common plants that are hazardous in your region:

The symptoms of plant poisoning can be extremely diverse, ranging from nausea and vomiting to rashes on the skin and even organ failure in extreme cases.

Identification: Attempt to ascertain the plant's identity in order to learn more about the probable toxins it contains. This information can help direct treatment.

Decontamination: Activated charcoal and other decontamination methods should be considered in the event that the substance was ingested. In the event of skin contact, the afflicted area should be washed carefully.

Care That Is Supportive It is important to provide care that is supportive for the patient depending on their symptoms and the specific toxins that are present.

Incidents Involving Dangerous Materials (also Known as "Hazmat")

There is a possibility that paramedics will respond to situations involving hazardous materials, which may involve the release of chemicals, gases, or other potentially harmful substances:

Safety at the Scene: In order to guarantee the safety of the scene, you must first determine the hazardous materials that are there and the possible dangers that they pose to both first responders and the general public.

Protective Gear It is important to wear the appropriate personal protective equipment (PPE) in order to reduce the likelihood of being exposed to potentially harmful substances.

Decontamination: Decontaminate patients who have been exposed to harmful contaminants as quickly as feasible in order to stop any additional damage from occurring.

In the event of a hazardous materials incident, the priority may shift from providing definitive care to stabilizing patients receiving advanced life support. Getting patients to a hospital or other medical facility as quickly as possible is frequently a top concern.

It is essential to perform round-the-clock surveillance of patients to look for any symptoms of chemical exposure and to assess their general state.

Marine Animals Can Cause Severe Bites and Stings

The dangers that come with being in an aquatic environment are one of a kind. Concerning the treatment of bites and stings:

Envenomation by Marine Life Envenomation can be caused by a variety of marine animals, including jellyfish, stingrays, and sea urchins. Locate the animal in question and administer the necessary first aid procedures after doing so.

Shark Bites Shark bites are extremely uncommon but can cause catastrophic harm if they do occur. Maintain the patient's stability, stop the bleeding, and start advanced trauma care only if it's necessary.

When treating bites and stings from marine animals, it is imperative that the safety of both the patient and the responders be prioritized at all times.

Illness Caused by Altitude

The symptoms of altitude sickness manifest themselves at high elevations and can strike anyone who ascend too quickly. The following are the primary manifestations of high-altitude illness:

Acute Mountain Sickness (AMS): AMS is the mildest form of acute mountain sickness and involves symptoms such as headache, nausea, and exhaustion. AMS sufferers may also experience a loss of appetite. Encourage relaxation and drinking plenty of water.

High-Altitude Pulmonary Edema (HAPE): HAPE is characterized by an accumulation of fluid in the lungs, which results in significant problems in breathing. As soon as possible, descend to lower altitudes and begin providing oxygen.

High-Altitude Cerebral Edema (HACE): High-Altitude Cerebral Edema causes swelling in the brain and is a disorder that can be fatal. In addition to receiving supportive care, rapid descent is necessary.

Educate patients about acclimatization and the importance of avoiding quick ascents as one of the preventative measures. Take it slow and be alert of the warning symptoms of high-altitude disease as you ascend.

Exposition to Radiation

Radiation exposure can be caused by a variety of factors, such as receiving medical treatment, being involved in an industrial disaster, or experiencing a nuclear catastrophe. Consider the following important factors:

Decontamination: If there is any reason to assume that the patient has been exposed to radiation, decontaminating them is necessary to stop the spread of radioactive material.

Patients should be categorized into groups according to the amount of radiation to which they have been exposed, and then care should be administered accordingly. The focus should be on activities that save lives.

Radiation Sickness: Be ready to detect the symptoms of radiation sickness and provide supportive care for those affected by this condition, which can result in nausea, vomiting, and suppression of bone marrow.

Isolation and Protection: In order to stop any future radiation exposure, patients who may have been contaminated with radioactive material should be isolated and protected.

Urgent Matters in the Wilderness

Those who serve as paramedics in wilderness or other isolated locations need to be ready for certain very specific challenges:

Access: The location of wilderness incidents, as well as how easily they may be reached, can be a source of difficulty. Make sure you are well-prepared to perform any necessary rescues or evacuations.

Hydration and Nutrition It is possible for patients to become dehydrated or malnourished after being exposed to the elements for an extended period of time. Don't forget to provide them hydration and food as needed.

The exposure to cold temperatures that might be found in wilderness settings can cause hypothermia. Patients should be gently rewarmed, and subsequent complications should be monitored.

Animal Encounters Patients may have had direct or indirect contact with wild animals, which could have resulted in physical harm or an infection. Evaluate, and then manage things correctly.

Risks of Infection: Wounds or contact with contaminated water can both put patients at risk for infections. Infections should be avoided and treated as required.

Advanced Life Support is covered in Chapter 17.

Paramedics play a vital role in the delivery of advanced medical interventions to patients who are in critical circumstances and are responsible for providing Advanced Life Support (ALS), which is an essential component of pre-hospital care. This chapter looks into the ideas, processes, and equipment used in Advanced Life Support. It covers a variety of topics, including the management of airways, the administration of medications, cardiac care, and other topics.

A Comprehensive Overview of Advanced Life Support

complex Life Support (ALS) is a level of pre-hospital treatment that involves complex medical procedures, interventions, and the administration of drugs by paramedics. This level of care is the highest level of care that can be provided outside of a hospital. ALS providers are healthcare professionals who have received extensive training and are able to undertake a broad variety of medical tasks that go beyond the interventions of Basic Life Support (BLS).

The basic objectives of the ALS program are to:

Patients who are seriously ill or injured need to be stabilized and managed.

Improve the patient's outcome by giving them their prescribed medications and treatments.

Offer more sophisticated management of the airways and ventilation.

Perform close observation and analysis of all vital signs, including readings from electrocardiograms (ECGs).

Getting patients ready for the right medical institutions and transporting them there.

Management of the Airway

Patients with compromised airways or patients who are unable to maintain their airway independently are the most likely to benefit from effective airway management. This is because effective airway management ensures that patients receive appropriate oxygenation and ventilation. A patent airway can be secured and maintained with the help of a variety of techniques and pieces of equipment used by ALS providers.

Manual Airway Maneuvers The head-tilt-chin-lift and jaw-thrust techniques are two of the fundamental manual airway maneuvers that can be used to open the airway depending on the state of the patient and the possibility of a cervical spine injury.

Supraglottic Airways: Supraglottic airway devices, such as the laryngeal mask airway (LMA) and the King Airway, are helpful tools for maintaining an airway in patients who may not require endotracheal intubation. These patients are referred to as "non-endotracheal candidates."

Endotracheal Intubation ALS caregivers receive training in endotracheal intubation, a procedure that involves inserting a tube into the trachea of the patient in order to secure the airway. This is absolutely necessary in situations where there is a severe obstruction of the airway, such as in individuals who have suffered serious head trauma or are unable to breathe.

Cricothyrotomy: A cricothyrotomy is a procedure that is performed to create an emergency airway through the cricothyroid membrane. This procedure is only used in exceptional circumstances where standard intubation cannot be performed.

Care for the Heart

Because of the frequency with which paramedics are dispatched to address cardiac arrest, chest discomfort, and arrhythmias, cardiac care is an essential component of ALS. The following are important components:

CPR, or cardiopulmonary resuscitation, is a lifesaving technique that must be performed immediately after a cardiac arrest and with as few breaks as possible. During cardiopulmonary resuscitation (CPR), paramedics utilize cutting-edge defibrillators and monitor ECG rhythms.

Defibrillation: Emergency medical technicians evaluate and treat shockable rhythms using automated external defibrillators, also known as AEDs. These rhythms include ventricular fibrillation and ventricular tachycardia.

drugs: During the management of cardiac arrest and arrhythmias, ALS providers deliver drugs such as epinephrine, amiodarone, and lidocaine.

12-Lead Electrocardiogram: Paramedics use 12-lead ECGs to look for alterations in the ST-segment, which can be a sign of myocardial infarction (also known as a heart attack).

Pacing: Patients who have bradycardia or heart blockages that do not respond to medicines may be candidates for transcutaneous pacing.

Advanced ECG Interpretation: Paramedics receive training that enables them to identify conditions that pose a hazard to life and interpret various ECG rhythms.

The Administration of Medication

A variety of drugs, including those used to treat pain, heart disorders, respiratory distress, and other medical difficulties, can be administered by medical professionals who provide ALS. The following are examples of common drugs that are prescribed:

Epinephrine is a drug that is administered to patients who are experiencing a cardiac arrest or severe allergic responses (anaphylaxis).

A bronchodilator that is used to treat asthma and other respiratory conditions is called albuterol.

Naloxone is used to reverse the effects of an opioid overdose.

Patients who are thought to be having a heart attack are often prescribed aspirin to prevent the formation of blood clots.

Nitroglycerin is a vasodilator that is also used to relieve chest pain while treating diseases related to the heart.

Glucose is a type of sugar that is given to people who have hypoglycemia (low blood sugar).

Adenosine is a drug that is administered to patients suffering from specific types of arrhythmias, including supraventricular tachycardia (SVT).

The Management of Trauma

Providers of ALS are trained and equipped to treat catastrophic injuries, including the following:

Controlling Hemorrhaging involves applying tourniquets, pressure dressings, and other hemostatic substances in order to stem the flow of blood.

Chest decompression refers to the process of placing a chest decompression needle in order to relieve tension pneumothorax.

Plaster casts are used to immobilize broken bones and dislocated joints to alleviate pain and prevent future injury.

Evaluation: In order to determine which injuries pose the greatest risk to the patient's life and to establish a treatment order, a comprehensive trauma evaluation is performed.

Emergencies Related to the Nervous System

The following are some examples of neurological emergencies that paramedics are trained to recognize and manage:

Stroke care involves recognizing the warning signs of a stroke and getting the patient to a stroke center as quickly as possible.

Seizures require the administration of drugs to control the patient's breathing and halt the seizures.

Assessing head injuries and keeping an eye out for any changes in neurological status is part of the treatment for head trauma.

Immobilizing patients suspected of having spinal cord injuries and controlling neurological impairments are two aspects of treating spinal cord injuries.

Emergencies Related to the Lungs and the Throat

The following strategies are used by ALS providers to manage respiratory distress and pulmonary conditions:

Oxygen therapy is the practice of administering supplementary oxygen in order to keep the patient's oxygen saturation levels at an adequate level.

The use of bag-valve-mask (BVM) ventilation or mechanical ventilators to assist patients who are unable to adequately breathe on their own is referred to as ventilatory support.

The management of patients who present with chest pain, shortness of breath, and a possible cardiac or respiratory disorder is referred to as chest pain and dyspnea.

Recognizing pneumothorax and treating chest trauma are both important aspects of pneumothorax management.

Emergencies Related to the Endocrine and Metabolic Systems

Emergency medical technicians often deal with endocrine and metabolic crises, such as the following:

Treatment of diabetic patients suffering from hyperglycemia or hypoglycemia, including the administration of glucose or insulin as required in the event of an emergency involving diabetes.

Electrolyte Imbalances: The management of conditions associated to electrolyte imbalances, including sodium, potassium, and calcium.

Recognizing and managing individuals who are experiencing adrenal crises is essential in treating adrenal insufficiency.

Urgences Relating to the Digestive System

The following are some of the ways that paramedics respond to gastrointestinal emergencies:

The treatment of nausea and vomiting involves giving antiemetic drugs to the patient in order to alleviate their symptoms.

Bleeding from the Gastrointestinal Tract Management of patients suffering from gastrointestinal bleeding and evaluation for shock.

Assessing and treating people who are suffering from stomach pain while taking into account the underlying reasons of this condition is known as abdominal pain management.

Infectious Diseases and Their Connections to the Environment

Patients with infectious infections and environmental exposures can be managed by ALS providers in the following ways:

When dealing with infectious diseases, it is important to take infection prevention steps and recognize the importance of isolating potentially infected individuals.

Toxic Exposures: The management of patients who have been exposed to potentially harmful substances, radiation, or materials.

Preparedness for and response to infectious disease outbreaks, including occurrences involving large numbers of casualties. Infectious Disease Outbreaks.

Emergencies of a Psychological and Behavioral Nature

In their training, paramedics learn how to manage patients who are experiencing psychological and behavioral emergencies, such as the following:

Managing patients who are irritated or violent in a safe manner is the topic of this unit.

Assessing patients who have suicidal ideation and taking the necessary precautions to ensure their safety is what we mean when we talk about suicidal ideation.

Abuse of Substances: The provision of medical assistance to patients who are under the influence of alcohol or narcotics, including the administration of medication such as naloxone in the event of an opioid overdose.

Recognizing the warning signals of domestic abuse and making sure victims are kept safe are two important aspects of this issue.

Certain Groups of People

The following are some examples of the demographics for which paramedics are trained to provide specialized care:

Pediatric amyotrophic lateral sclerosis (ALS) entails taking into account the specific requirements of pediatric patients and adjusting treatment accordingly.

Geriatric ALS refers to the administration of proper care to aged patients, taking into account their comorbidities as well as their drugs.

Patients Who Are Pregnant: Taking care of pregnant patients and responding to obstetric situations such as labor that begins too early.

Patients with Disabilities: Ensuring Accessible and Culturally Competent Care for Patients With Physical, Sensory, Intellectual, or Developmental Disabilities Patients with disabilities include those who have physical, sensory, intellectual, or developmental impairments.

A Look at Some Ethical Considerations Regarding ALS

In ALS, paramedics are required to manage a complicated set of ethical considerations, including the following:

Respecting patients' advance directives, do-not-resuscitate (DNR), and medical power of attorney orders is an important part of providing good medical care.

End-of-Life Care: The practice of providing patients and their families with compassionate end-of-life care, which may include palliative care and emotional support.

Informed permission refers to the process of ensuring that patients or their legal representatives provide informed permission for medical interventions whenever it is practicable to do so.

Patient autonomy refers to the practice of respecting patient autonomy and include patients in decision-making regarding their care whenever it is practicable to do so.

Continuing Education as well as Certification Retests

ALS paramedics are required to participate in continual education and training in order to keep their skills up to date and remain knowledgeable of the most effective methods and most recent medical protocols. The procedures for re-certification can vary from region to region, but they typically consist of periodical evaluations of one's skills as well as written and oral examinations.

Systems for Treating Trauma Patients and Triage

When it comes to providing the best possible care and results for injured patients, trauma systems and efficient triage play an essential role. The organization of trauma systems, the concepts of trauma triage, and the methods that guide paramedics in identifying and prioritizing patients in need of urgent care are all covered in depth in this chapter.

An Overview of Different Trauma Systems

Trauma systems are all-encompassing and well-organized methods for providing the best possible care to people who have been injured. They make use of a network of healthcare institutions, ranging from pre-hospital care to trauma centers, in order to guarantee that patients who have suffered trauma receive care that is prompt and appropriate. The following are the primary elements that make up trauma systems:

Care Provided Before Admission to a Hospital Pre-hospital care is provided by paramedics and other members of emergency medical services (EMS), who are the initial point of contact for trauma victims. They are responsible for providing initial assessments, bringing the patient to a stable state, and transporting them to the right facility.

Trauma Centers A trauma center is a specialist hospital that possesses the resources and the experience necessary to give decisive care to patients who have sustained catastrophic injuries. On the basis of their capabilities and resources, they are placed into one of four different levels: I, II, III, or IV.

Emergency Departments: General emergency departments also play a role in trauma care because they receive a variety of patients and stabilize those who have injuries before transferring them to trauma centers. This is done before the patients are taken to trauma centers.

Rehabilitation Services: Trauma systems typically offer rehabilitation services, which aim to assist patients in recovering from their injuries and regaining their functional capacities.

Both the prevention of traumatic events and the education of the general public are essential components of trauma systems. This is because the incidence of traumatic events should be reduced as much as possible.

Data and the Improvement of Quality Trauma systems collect data on the outcomes of their patients and utilize this information to improve the quality of the care they provide. This strategy, which is data-driven, helps discover areas that could use some work.

The Principles of Trauma Triage

The process of identifying and prioritizing injured patients in the event of a trauma is referred to as "trauma triage," and it is dependent on the severity of the patients' injuries and the resources that are available. An efficient trauma triage system guarantees that patients receive the right care even as it keeps medical facilities from becoming overwhelmed. The following are the core tenets of trauma triage:

The mechanism of injury is evaluated by the paramedics, who take into consideration a variety of criteria that may include the patient's ejection from the car, the type of contact, and the vehicle's speed. Mechanisms requiring a lot of energy could be an indication of a severe injury.

Physiological Criteria The evaluation of the patient's vital signs and degree of consciousness are required in order to satisfy the physiological criteria. Important parameters include the patient's heart rate, blood pressure, breathing rate, and their score on the Glasgow Coma Scale (GCS).

Anatomic Criteria: The anatomic criteria place an emphasis on particular injuries or conditions, such as open fractures, serious head injuries, or injuries that have the potential to affect the airway, respiration, or circulation.

Taking Special Into Account: When taking special considerations, it is important to take into account the patient's age, any comorbid conditions they may have, as well as whether or not they are pregnant.

Time Spent in Transport: The amount of time it takes to go to a trauma center is an essential component to consider when deciding where the patient will be taken.

Categories for Use in Triage

Patients who have been exposed to trauma are often placed into one of the following tiers based on the severity of their injuries:

Patients classified as imminent have sustained injuries that pose an immediate risk to their lives and require prompt medical attention. They are the highest priority, and they need to be taken to a trauma center as soon as it is possible to do so.

Patients that are considered to be in an emergency situation have suffered critical injuries that require immediate medical attention, but they are stable enough to be able to bear a little delay in transportation. They need to be taken to an emergency room or another hospital that is equipped to do surgery as soon as possible.

Urgent patients have substantial injuries, but they are stable enough to tolerate a lengthier wait in transport. Urgent patients are taken to the hospital as quickly as possible. They should be taken by ambulance to a facility that is suitable for the kind of harm they have sustained.

Patients that are classified as non-urgent have injuries that do not pose an immediate threat to their lives, and as a result, their transportation can be delayed even further. They need to be evaluated and treated in the right facility, which they should be taken to.

Protocols for the Management of Trauma

Protocols for trauma triage are typically defined at the regional or state level, and these protocols guide the decision-making process for paramedics and other healthcare workers. When evaluating patients with trauma, particular criteria and procedures have to be followed, as outlined in the protocol. These protocols are derived from evidence-based principles and are continually revised to reflect the most recent developments in industry standards.

The following are typical components of protocols for trauma triage:

The Field Triage Decision Scheme is a decision guide that assists paramedics in classifying patients according to the clinical status of the patients and the manner in which they were injured.

The protocols decide which facility will be used as the triage patient's final destination for each of the categories of patients. This may include emergency rooms, trauma centers, or other specialist medical institutions.

Criteria for Skipping Hospitals Patients may be skipped over in certain circumstances in order to ensure that they are treated at the institution that is best suited to their needs rather than first going to a nearby hospital.

Air Medical Transport: Protocols may include criteria for air medical transport, which is critical for the expeditious transportation of seriously injured patients to trauma centers.

Guidelines for moving patients from one hospital to another promote continuity of care and keep track of the patient's triage status. These transfers are referred to as "interfacility transfers."

Data Collection and Reporting Collection and reporting of data on trauma patients, including triage categories and outcomes, is frequently required by protocols.

Incidents with Multiple Casualties That Require Triage

Protocols for trauma triage are also applicable in the event of mass casualty occurrences (MCIs), which can include both natural and man-made disasters, as well as industrial accidents and terrorist attacks. In these kinds of scenarios, paramedics are faced with the difficult task of evaluating a large number of injured patients and determining which ones are most urgent. During the MCI triage process, key considerations include:

Safety at the Scene: It is of the utmost importance to guarantee the safety of first responders as well as any subsequent victims.

Establishing a system for the rapid triage of patients via color-coded tags or other approaches may be referred to as "Rapid Triage."

Patients are placed into one of four basic categories throughout the triage process. These categories are immediate, delayed, minimal, and expectant.

The process of continually reassessing patients and modifying their triage categories as their diseases progress is referred to as "reassessment."

The process of dividing up limited resources, such as personnel and medical supplies, in order to meet the most pressing requirements first is known as resource allocation.

Transportation: coordinating transportation in order to guarantee that patients are transported to the most suitable institutions in the most time-effective manner.

Triage of Pediatric Patients

When triaging pediatric patients, there are several specific considerations that need to be made because children may appear differently than adults and have different physiological responses to trauma. Triage in pediatrics may involve the following:

Age-Based Criteria In order to properly classify pediatric patients, triage protocols may include age-based criteria. These criteria acknowledge the fact that newborns, children, and adolescents have distinct physiological reactions to trauma.

Considerations Relating to Children's Development Understanding the requirements and actions of children requires that paramedics evaluate the children's developmental stage.

Assessment of Pain: Evaluating a patient's level of discomfort by applying techniques that are tailored to the patient's age group.

Family Presence refers to the act of offering emotional support to both the child and their family as well as involving the child's parents or guardians in the triage process.

Equipment Tailored Specifically for Children Ensuring the Availability of Equipment Tailored Specifically for Children This includes Airway Management Equipment and Medication Administration Equipment.

During the triage process, creating a setting that is child-friendly can help lessen anxious feelings and tension for both patients and their families.

Triage of Geriatric Patients

Patients of any age require specialized triage considerations, but elderly patients in particular do so since they frequently have several comorbidities and specific requirements:

Conducting a thorough assessment in order to identify subtle injuries and concomitant conditions that might not be immediately apparent is what is meant by the term "comprehensive assessment."

Considerations Regarding Medication This includes being aware of the possibility of interactions between medications as well as age-related changes in how drugs are metabolized.

Evaluation of frailty includes determining whether or not a person is frail and modifying care to account for functional limitations and cognitive shifts.

Palliative care and end-of-life conversations involve having conversations with elderly patients about their end-of-life choices and options for palliative care while respecting the patients' autonomy and personal preferences.

During an outbreak of an infectious disease, triage is performed.

Patients who have been injured may be afflicted with highly dangerous infections, which presents a special set of issues for the triage process used in trauma centers. Pandemics are one type of infectious disease epidemic. During epidemics of infectious diseases, some important things to keep in mind include:

Implementing Strict Infection Control Measures The implementation of stringent infection control measures is necessary to safeguard both patients and healthcare providers.

Establishing Triage Facilities: Establishing triage facilities that are specifically designed for the screening and isolation of infectious diseases.

Personal Protective Equipment (PPE): Ensuring that paramedics and healthcare personnel have access to and are using the appropriate PPE at all times.

Protocols for Quarantine and Isolation: Adhering to protocols for quarantine and isolation for patients who may be infected, while also providing the essential care to these patients.

Assessment of Risk: Continually evaluating the potential for contamination with infectious illnesses and modifying triage and treatment processes in accordance with the findings.

Ethical Considerations in the Treatment of Trauma Victims

When there are limited resources available or several patients that need rapid care at the same time, it is very important to keep ethical considerations in mind while doing trauma triage. Principles of ethics include the following:

The invention and deployment of evidence-based algorithms for the purpose of ensuring fairness and consistency in triage judgments is referred to as "triage algorithms."

When making triage decisions, non-discrimination means not giving preference to patients based on characteristics like as age, gender, race, religion, or handicap.

Transparency refers to the practice of conveying triage decisions and criteria to patients and their families in an open and honest manner whenever this is possible.

When making decisions on triage, including those regarding end-of-life care, it is important to respect the patients' right to autonomy as well as their wishes.

The act of giving priority to decisions that are in the patient's and the larger community's best interests is known as beneficence.

Justice is the process of allocating resources in a manner that is just and equitable, taking into account what is in the patients' best interests as a whole.

Practice Questions and Answers Explanations 2023-2024

Question 1:
A patient presents with confusion, severe respiratory distress, and an oxygen saturation of 87%. What should you suspect, and what is the initial treatment?

A) Pulmonary embolism; administer oxygen and perform rapid sequence intubation.
B) Acute asthma exacerbation; administer nebulized albuterol and oxygen.
C) Myocardial infarction; administer aspirin and nitroglycerin.
D) Anaphylactic shock; administer epinephrine and an antihistamine.

Answer 1:
B) Acute asthma exacerbation; administer nebulized albuterol and oxygen.

Explanation 1:
The patient's symptoms and low oxygen saturation are indicative of an acute asthma exacerbation. The initial treatment should focus on improving airflow and oxygenation, making option B the correct choice.

Question 2:
During a trauma call, a patient presents with decerebrate posturing, fixed and dilated pupils, and abnormal respirations. What injury is most likely responsible?

A) Basilar skull fracture
B) Epidural hematoma
C) Hypoxic brain injury
D) Cerebral contusion

Answer 2:
B) Epidural hematoma

Explanation 2:
The presentation of decerebrate posturing, fixed and dilated pupils, and abnormal respirations suggests a severe brain injury, which is often seen with an epidural hematoma.

Question 3:
What is the primary purpose of the Glasgow Coma Scale (GCS)?

A) To assess vital signs in trauma patients.
B) To evaluate the level of consciousness in patients with head injuries.
C) To measure oxygen saturation in patients with respiratory distress.
D) To calculate the Injury Severity Score (ISS) in trauma patients.

Answer 3:
B) To evaluate the level of consciousness in patients with head injuries.

Explanation 3:
The GCS is a tool used to assess a patient's level of consciousness, especially in those with head injuries. It helps quantify a patient's neurological status.

Question 4:
What is the most appropriate treatment for a patient in ventricular fibrillation?

A) Administer a 12-lead ECG.
B) Perform synchronized cardioversion.
C) Administer epinephrine.
D) Defibrillate with a biphasic defibrillator.

Answer 4:
D) Defibrillate with a biphasic defibrillator.

Explanation 4:
Ventricular fibrillation is a life-threatening arrhythmia that requires immediate defibrillation. Use a biphasic defibrillator to deliver an electrical shock to the heart.

Question 5:
You arrive at the scene of a motor vehicle accident. The patient is unconscious, has slow and shallow breathing, and is trapped in the vehicle. What is your first action?

A) Administer high-flow oxygen.
B) Apply cervical spine immobilization.
C) Perform a rapid extrication.
D) Request a helicopter for immediate transport.

Answer 5:
B) Apply cervical spine immobilization.

Explanation 5:
The patient's condition, mechanism of injury, and the need for extrication indicate the importance of cervical spine immobilization before any other intervention.

Question 6:
A patient with a traumatic amputation of the arm is bleeding profusely. What is the initial treatment priority?

A) Elevate the residual limb.
B) Apply a tourniquet proximal to the injury.
C) Administer pain medication.
D) Apply a pressure dressing.

Answer 6:
B) Apply a tourniquet proximal to the injury.

Explanation 6:
In cases of profuse bleeding from a traumatic amputation, applying a tourniquet proximal to the injury is the primary treatment to control bleeding.

Question 7:
A 55-year-old patient presents with chest pain radiating to the left arm, diaphoresis, and shortness of breath. Which medication is most appropriate to administer?

A) Epinephrine
B) Nitroglycerin
C) Albuterol
D) Aspirin

Answer 7:
D) Aspirin

Explanation 7:
The patient's symptoms are consistent with a myocardial infarction. Administering aspirin helps reduce platelet aggregation and should be given promptly.

Question 8:
A patient is experiencing an acute allergic reaction with severe difficulty breathing and hypotension. What is the initial treatment of choice?

A) Epinephrine
B) Albuterol
C) Nitroglycerin
D) Furosemide

Answer 8:
A) Epinephrine

Explanation 8:
In cases of anaphylaxis, epinephrine is the primary treatment to counteract severe allergic reactions, improve breathing, and raise blood pressure.

Question 9:
You are assessing a pediatric patient who is experiencing stridor, drooling, and tripod positioning. What is the most likely diagnosis?

A) Asthma exacerbation
B) Croup (laryngotracheobronchitis)
C) Epiglottitis
D) Bronchiolitis

Answer 9:
C) Epiglottitis

Explanation 9:
Stridor, drooling, and tripod positioning are classic signs of epiglottitis, a potentially life-threatening condition that requires immediate medical attention.

Question 10:
Which of the following patients is most at risk for heat-related illnesses during a hot summer day?

A) A construction worker who is well-hydrated.
B) An elderly woman with a history of heatstroke.
C) A teenager playing basketball outdoors with friends.
D) An office worker who occasionally takes breaks outside.

Answer 10:
B) An elderly woman with a history of heatstroke.

Explanation 10:
Elderly individuals, especially those with a history of heat-related illnesses, are at a higher risk for heat-related illnesses due to their decreased ability to regulate body temperature.

Question 11:
A patient presents with pinpoint pupils, respiratory depression, and altered mental status. Which substance is most likely responsible?

A) Opioids
B) Benzodiazepines
C) Amphetamines
D) Cocaine

Answer 11:
A) Opioids

Explanation 11:
Pinpoint pupils, respiratory depression, and altered mental status are classic signs of opioid overdose.

Question 12:
What is the first-line treatment for a patient with a suspected tension pneumothorax?

A) Administer high-flow oxygen.
B) Perform needle decompression.
C) Apply an occlusive dressing.
D) Administer bronchodilators.

Answer 12:
B) Perform needle decompression.

Explanation 12:
A tension pneumothorax is a life-threatening condition that requires immediate decompression. The treatment of choice is needle decompression.

Question 13:
You are called to a motor vehicle accident involving a pregnant woman. She is in her third trimester, and the vehicle was struck from behind. The patient is experiencing abdominal pain and contractions. What is the most likely concern?

A) Placental abruption
B) Uterine rupture
C) Preterm labor
D) Shoulder dystocia

Answer 13:
A) Placental abruption

Explanation 13:
In a pregnant woman with abdominal pain and contractions after a motor vehicle accident, the concern is a placental abruption, which can lead to severe bleeding and fetal distress.

Question 14:
Which of the following injuries requires immediate surgical intervention and cannot be managed in the pre-hospital setting?

A) Open femur fracture
B) Abdominal evisceration
C) Closed head injury
D) Flail chest

Answer 14:
B) Abdominal evisceration

Explanation 14:
Abdominal evisceration, where the abdominal contents are exposed, is a surgical emergency and cannot be managed in the pre-hospital setting.

Question 15:
A patient is experiencing severe epistaxis (nosebleed) with ongoing bleeding. What is the most appropriate action?

A) Pinch the patient's nose and have them lean forward.
B) Have the patient lie flat on their back.
C) Apply ice packs to the patient's neck.
D) Administer nasal decongestant spray.

Answer 15:
A) Pinch the patient's nose and have them lean forward.

Explanation 15:
For severe epistaxis, the patient should pinch their nose and lean forward to prevent blood from flowing down the throat and into the stomach.

Question 16:
A patient with a history of hypertension is experiencing a severe headache, visual disturbances, and weakness on one side of their body. What condition should you suspect?

A) Migraine
B) Hemorrhagic stroke
C) Tension headache
D) Sinusitis

Answer 16:
B) Hemorrhagic stroke

Explanation 16:
The patient's symptoms, including a severe headache and neurological deficits, are consistent with a hemorrhagic stroke, which is associated with hypertension.

Question 17:
You are assessing a patient who has been exposed to a hazardous chemical. What is the first step in managing chemical exposures?

A) Decontaminate the patient.
B) Administer an antidote.
C) Apply an occlusive dressing.
D) Initiate positive-pressure ventilation.

Answer 17:
A) Decontaminate the patient.

Explanation 17:
In cases of chemical exposure, the first step is to decontaminate the patient to prevent further harm or contamination.

Question 18:
A patient with diabetes presents with altered mental status, rapid breathing, and a fruity odor on their breath. What condition is most likely responsible for these findings?

A) Hypoglycemia
B) Hyperglycemia (diabetic ketoacidosis)
C) Stroke
D) Sepsis

Answer 18:
B) Hyperglycemia (diabetic ketoacidosis)

Explanation 18:
The patient's altered mental status, rapid breathing, and fruity odor on their breath are indicative of hyperglycemia, specifically diabetic ketoacidosis.

Question 19:
A patient has fallen from a significant height and presents with abdominal pain, guarding, and ecchymosis (bruising) around the umbilicus. What is the likely diagnosis?

A) Renal colic
B) Abdominal aortic aneurysm
C) Blunt abdominal trauma
D) Appendicitis

Answer 19:
C) Blunt abdominal trauma

Explanation 19:
The patient's history and symptoms suggest blunt abdominal trauma, which can lead to internal injuries, including the rupture of abdominal organs or vessels.

Question 20:
A patient with a history of epilepsy is experiencing a seizure. What is the most appropriate action?

A) Place an object in the patient's mouth to prevent them from biting their tongue.
B) Restrain the patient to prevent injury.
C) Protect the patient from injury by moving objects away and placing them on their side.
D) Administer an antipsychotic medication.

Answer 20:
C) Protect the patient from injury by moving objects away and placing them on their side.

Explanation 20:
During a seizure, the primary goal is to protect the patient from injury by moving objects away and placing them on their side. Do not place objects in the patient's mouth, and do not restrain them.

Question 21:
A patient is experiencing a suspected overdose on benzodiazepines. What is the appropriate treatment?

A) Administer naloxone.
B) Provide intravenous glucose.
C) Administer flumazenil.
D) Initiate positive-pressure ventilation.

Answer 21:
C) Administer flumazenil.

Explanation 21:
Flumazenil is the specific antidote for benzodiazepine overdoses and should be administered if the overdose is suspected.

Question 22:
What is the primary concern when treating a patient with a severe burn injury?

A) Infection control
B) Pain management
C) Oxygen administration
D) Splinting the burn area

Answer 22:
A) Infection control

Explanation 22:
Infection control is the primary concern in treating severe burn injuries. Burns expose the patient to a high risk of infection, and measures should be taken to prevent and manage infection.

Question 23:
You are treating a patient with severe hypothermia. What is the most appropriate method to rewarm the patient?

A) Apply a heating pad directly to the skin.
B) Immerse the patient in hot water.
C) Use passive external rewarming techniques.
D) Administer hot beverages intravenously.

Answer 23:
C) Use passive external rewarming techniques.

Explanation 23:
Passive external rewarming, such as providing warm blankets and shelter, is the preferred method for rewarming a severely hypothermic patient. Direct heat application or hot water immersion can cause further harm.

Question 24:
A patient presents with sudden-onset chest pain, pleuritic in nature, and associated with shortness of breath. Which condition should you suspect?

A) Myocardial infarction
B) Pneumothorax
C) Pulmonary embolism
D) Aortic dissection

Answer 24:
C) Pulmonary embolism

Explanation 24:
Sudden-onset pleuritic chest pain and shortness of breath are classic symptoms of a pulmonary embolism, which is a blockage in the pulmonary artery.

Question 25:
You are treating a patient with a suspected spinal cord injury. What is the most appropriate way to immobilize the spine?

A) Place the patient in a Trendelenburg position.
B) Apply a rigid cervical collar.
C) Administer a muscle relaxant.
D) Keep the patient supine without any immobilization.

Answer 25:
B) Apply a rigid cervical collar.

Explanation 25:

In cases of a suspected spinal cord injury, it is essential to immobilize the spine. This is typically done by applying a rigid cervical collar and using a backboard or similar device for full spinal immobilization.

Question 26:
A 6-month-old infant is unresponsive and not breathing. What is the initial action you should take?

A) Administer 2 rescue breaths.
B) Begin CPR with chest compressions.
C) Start with abdominal thrusts.
D) Elevate the infant's legs.

Answer 26:
B) Begin CPR with chest compressions.

Explanation 26:
For infants, if they are unresponsive and not breathing, the initial action is to begin CPR with chest compressions. This is because cardiac arrest is the most likely cause of the symptoms.

Question 27:
A patient presents with slurred speech, facial droop, and weakness on one side of their body. What condition should you suspect?

A) Seizure
B) Hypoglycemia
C) Stroke
D) Anxiety

Answer 27:
C) Stroke

Explanation 27:
The patient's symptoms are indicative of a stroke, specifically a neurological deficit.

Question 28:
You are called to the scene of a motorcycle crash. The rider is wearing a helmet and has a Glasgow Coma Scale (GCS) score of 15. What is the most appropriate action?

A) Apply a cervical collar and backboard.
B) Request a helicopter for immediate transport.
C) Administer high-flow oxygen.
D) Conduct a rapid extrication.

Answer 28:
C) Administer high-flow oxygen.

Explanation 28:
With a GCS score of 15, the patient's airway and breathing are likely intact. Administering high-flow oxygen is appropriate for a motorcycle crash patient.

Question 29:
A patient with a history of chronic obstructive pulmonary disease (COPD) presents with severe shortness of breath, cyanosis, and the use of accessory muscles for breathing. What is the initial treatment?

A) Administer nitroglycerin.
B) Administer nebulized albuterol.
C) Perform synchronized cardioversion.
D) Administer epinephrine.

Answer 29:
B) Administer nebulized albuterol.

Explanation 29:
The patient's presentation is consistent with a COPD exacerbation. The initial treatment is nebulized albuterol to improve airway function.

Question 30:
A patient presents with a 12-lead ECG showing ST-segment elevation in multiple leads. What is the likely diagnosis?

A) Sinus tachycardia
B) Ventricular fibrillation
C) Acute myocardial infarction
D) Atrial fibrillation

Answer 30:
C) Acute myocardial infarction

Explanation 30:
ST-segment elevation on a 12-lead ECG is indicative of an acute myocardial infarction (heart attack).

Question 31:
You arrive at a scene where a patient is trapped in a vehicle that has collided with a tree. The patient is responsive and alert but unable to move due to trapped legs. What is the priority in this situation?

A) Administer analgesics for pain.
B) Initiate extrication immediately.
C) Stabilize the cervical spine.
D) Administer high-flow oxygen.

Answer 31:
C) Stabilize the cervical spine.

Explanation 31:
In cases of motor vehicle accidents with potential trauma, it's essential to stabilize the cervical spine to prevent spinal cord injury before extrication.

Question 32:
A patient with a known penicillin allergy is experiencing an allergic reaction. What medication is the most appropriate treatment?

A) Diphenhydramine
B) Ceftriaxone
C) Aspirin
D) Prednisone

Answer 32:
A) Diphenhydramine

Explanation 32:
For an allergic reaction, especially with a known penicillin allergy, diphenhydramine is the appropriate treatment to relieve symptoms.

Question 33:
A patient with a gunshot wound to the abdomen is experiencing hypotension, tachycardia, and distended abdomen. What is the primary concern?

A) Hypoxia
B) Bleeding and hemorrhagic shock
C) Infection
D) Neurological deficit

Answer 33:
B) Bleeding and hemorrhagic shock

Explanation 33:
In a patient with a gunshot wound to the abdomen and signs of shock, the primary concern is bleeding and hemorrhagic shock.

Question 34:
A patient with severe dehydration may exhibit which clinical sign?

A) Bradycardia
B) Pale, cool, and clammy skin
C) Decreased urine output
D) Hypertension

Answer 34:
C) Decreased urine output

Explanation 34:
Decreased urine output is a clinical sign of severe dehydration, as the body conserves fluids.

Question 35:
You are treating a patient with a suspected opioid overdose. What is the first-line medication to administer?

A) Naloxone
B) Epinephrine
C) Diazepam
D) Albuterol

Answer 35:
A) Naloxone

Explanation 35:
Naloxone is the first-line medication for reversing opioid overdose by displacing opioids from receptor sites.

Question 36:
A patient with a traumatic brain injury presents with unequal pupils, altered mental status, and elevated blood pressure on one side. What type of injury should you suspect?

A) Concussion
B) Intracerebral hemorrhage
C) Epidural hematoma
D) Subdural hematoma

Answer 36:
C) Epidural hematoma

Explanation 36:
The presentation of unequal pupils, altered mental status, and elevated blood pressure on one side is indicative of an epidural hematoma, which is a collection of blood between the skull and the dura mater.

Question 37:
A patient with a severe burn injury is experiencing difficulty breathing. What condition should you suspect?

A) Hypovolemic shock
B) Inhalation injury
C) Cardiac tamponade
D) Hemorrhagic shock

Answer 37:
B) Inhalation injury

Explanation 37:
In patients with severe burn injuries and difficulty breathing, the concern is an inhalation injury caused by inhaling superheated air or toxic fumes.

Question 38:
A patient presents with a suspected spinal injury. What is the appropriate method for moving the patient to a backboard?

A) Place the patient in a lateral recumbent position and slide the board under them.
B) Roll the patient onto the board from their side.
C) Logroll the patient onto the board.
D) Lift the patient onto the board with the help of a second responder.

Answer 38:
C) Logroll the patient onto the board.

Explanation 38:
When moving a patient with a suspected spinal injury to a backboard, the logroll technique is used to maintain spinal alignment.

Question 39:
A 40-year-old male patient is experiencing chest pain and shortness of breath. He has a history of smoking and hypertension. What condition should you suspect?

A) Gastroesophageal reflux disease (GERD)
B) Anxiety attack
C) Myocardial infarction
D) Esophageal spasm

Answer 39:
C) Myocardial infarction

Explanation 39:
In a 40-year-old patient with chest pain, shortness of breath, and risk factors like smoking and hypertension, the concern is a myocardial infarction until ruled out.

Question 40:
You are treating a patient with a laceration on their arm. What is the appropriate method for wound irrigation?

A) Irrigate the wound with a saline solution.
B) Use hydrogen peroxide for wound irrigation.
C) Rinse the wound with warm, soapy water.
D) Apply a dry, sterile dressing without irrigation.

Answer 40:
A) Irrigate the wound with a saline solution.

Explanation 40:
The appropriate method for wound irrigation is to use a saline solution to remove debris and contaminants from the wound.

Question 41:
A patient presents with difficulty speaking, weakness on one side of their body, and a severe headache. What condition should you suspect?

A) Ischemic stroke
B) Tension headache
C) Migraine
D) Cluster headache

Answer 41:
A) Ischemic stroke

Explanation 41:
The patient's symptoms, including difficulty speaking, weakness, and a severe headache, are indicative of an ischemic stroke.

Question 42:
You are treating a patient with a suspected abdominal aortic aneurysm. What is the appropriate position for the patient?

A) Sitting upright
B) Lying flat on their back
C) Kneeling
D) In a semi-Fowler's position

Answer 42:
B) Lying flat on their back

Explanation 42:
In cases of a suspected abdominal aortic aneurysm, the patient should be placed in a supine position to reduce the risk of rupture.

Question 43:
You are assessing a patient with a traumatic head injury. What is a concerning finding related to their pupils?

A) Pupils that react to light and are equal in size
B) One dilated pupil and one constricted pupil
C) Pupils that are unequal but react to light
D) Fixed and dilated pupils

Answer 43:
D) Fixed and dilated pupils

Explanation 43:
Fixed and dilated pupils are concerning findings in a patient with a traumatic head injury and may indicate brain herniation.

Question 44:
A 25-year-old male is experiencing sudden-onset chest pain and shortness of breath. He has no significant medical history. What condition should you suspect?

A) A panic attack
B) Pulmonary embolism
C) Tension pneumothorax
D) Costochondritis

Answer 44:
B) Pulmonary embolism

Explanation 44:
In a young patient with sudden-onset chest pain and shortness of breath, the concern is a pulmonary embolism until ruled out.

Question 45:
You are treating a patient with a suspected fracture of the forearm. What is the appropriate method for splinting the injury?

A) Keep the arm immobilized against the patient's body.
B) Apply a rigid splint on one side of the arm.
C) Use pillows to support the injured arm.
D) Splint the arm to the chest.

Answer 45:
B) Apply a rigid splint on one side of the arm.

Explanation 45:
For a suspected forearm fracture, it's appropriate to apply a rigid splint on one side of the arm to immobilize the injury.

Question 46:
A patient presents with sudden-onset chest pain that radiates to the back, along with diaphoresis and nausea. What condition should you suspect?

A) Musculoskeletal chest pain
B) Acute gastritis
C) Aortic dissection
D) Gastroesophageal reflux disease (GERD)

Answer 46:
C) Aortic dissection

Explanation 46:
Sudden-onset chest pain radiating to the back, diaphoresis, and nausea are concerning symptoms of an aortic dissection, a life-threatening condition.

Question 47:
You are assessing a patient with a traumatic injury. What is the appropriate method for assessing the patient's circulation?

A) Check for pupillary reaction.
B) Assess the patient's level of consciousness.
C) Check peripheral pulses.
D) Observe chest rise and fall.

Answer 47:
C) Check peripheral pulses.

Explanation 47:
Assessing peripheral pulses is an appropriate method for evaluating a patient's circulation and perfusion status.

Question 48:
A 2-year-old child is experiencing stridor, retractions, and drooling. What is the likely diagnosis?

A) Asthma
B) Croup (laryngotracheobronchitis)
C) Epiglottitis
D) Bronchiolitis

Answer 48:
C) Epiglottitis

Explanation 48:
Stridor, retractions, and drooling in a child are classic signs of epiglottitis, a potentially life-threatening condition.

Question 49:
A patient with a suspected ankle fracture is unable to bear weight on the injured leg. What is the appropriate treatment?

A) Encourage the patient to walk to assess stability.
B) Apply a compression bandage.
C) Splint the ankle and assist with crutches.
D) Elevate the injured leg.

Answer 49:
C) Splint the ankle and assist with crutches.

Explanation 49:
In the case of a suspected ankle fracture, it is appropriate to splint the injury and assist the patient with crutches to prevent further damage.

Question 50:
You are treating a patient with severe hypothermia. What is the most appropriate method for rewarming the patient?

A) Apply heat packs to the patient's skin.
B) Immerse the patient in a hot bath.
C) Use active external rewarming techniques.
D) Administer hot fluids intravenously.

Answer 50:
C) Use active external rewarming techniques.

Explanation 50:
Active external rewarming techniques, such as using heated blankets or warm fluids, are appropriate for rewarming a severely hypothermic patient.

Question 51:
A patient presents with chest pain that worsens with deep breaths and is associated with fever. What condition should you suspect?

A) Myocardial infarction
B) Pneumothorax
C) Pneumonia
D) Rib fracture

Answer 51:
C) Pneumonia

Explanation 51:
Chest pain worsened by deep breaths and fever is indicative of a respiratory condition like pneumonia.

Question 52:
You are treating a pediatric patient who has ingested a household cleaning product. What is the appropriate initial action?

A) Induce vomiting to remove the toxin.
B) Administer activated charcoal.
C) Call the Poison Control Center.
D) Offer the child milk or water to dilute the substance.

Answer 52:
C) Call the Poison Control Center.

Explanation 52:
In cases of poison ingestion, the initial action is to call the Poison Control Center for guidance on appropriate management.

Question 53:
A patient presents with a weak and irregular pulse, rapid breathing, and altered mental status. What medication should you consider administering?

A) Atropine
B) Adenosine
C) Amiodarone
D) Epinephrine

Answer 53:
D) Epinephrine

Explanation 53:
The patient's presentation suggests a cardiac issue, and epinephrine is a medication that can help improve pulse and blood pressure.

Question 54:
A patient with a laceration on their leg is experiencing severe bleeding. What is the initial action?

A) Apply a tourniquet proximal to the injury.
B) Administer pain medication.
C) Elevate the patient's leg.
D) Apply direct pressure with a sterile dressing.

Answer 54:
D) Apply direct pressure with a sterile dressing.

Explanation 54:
In cases of severe bleeding, the initial action is to apply direct pressure with a sterile dressing to control the bleeding.

Question 55:
A patient with a history of heart failure is experiencing shortness of breath, pedal edema, and crackles in the lungs. What is the likely diagnosis?

A) Pneumonia
B) Congestive heart failure exacerbation
C) Pulmonary embolism
D) Pneumothorax

Answer 55:
B) Congestive heart failure exacerbation

Explanation 55:
The patient's symptoms, including shortness of breath, pedal edema, and lung crackles, are consistent with a congestive heart failure exacerbation.

Question 56:
A patient with a history of diabetes is experiencing altered mental status, hunger, and tremors. What condition should you suspect?

A) Hyperglycemia (diabetic ketoacidosis)
B) Hypoglycemia
C) Hyperthyroidism
D) Seizure

Answer 56:
B) Hypoglycemia

Explanation 56:
Altered mental status, hunger, and tremors are indicative of hypoglycemia, a common concern in patients with diabetes.

Question 57:
A patient with abdominal pain, nausea, and vomiting presents with a palpable mass in the lower-right abdomen. What condition should you suspect?

A) Gastroenteritis
B) Kidney stones
C) Appendicitis
D) Diverticulitis

Answer 57:
C) Appendicitis

Explanation 57:
A palpable mass in the lower-right abdomen, along with abdominal pain, nausea, and vomiting, is suggestive of appendicitis.

Question 58:
You are treating a patient with a suspected head injury. What is the appropriate method for controlling external bleeding?

A) Apply direct pressure to the wound.
B) Elevate the patient's head.
C) Administer an anticoagulant.
D) Use a tourniquet above the injury.

Answer 58:
A) Apply direct pressure to the wound.

Explanation 58:
For external bleeding in a patient with a head injury, the appropriate method is to apply direct pressure to the wound.

Question 59:
A patient is experiencing severe abdominal pain, distention, and absent bowel sounds. What condition should you suspect?

A) Constipation
B) Diverticulosis
C) Ileus
D) Appendicitis

Answer 59:
C) Ileus

Explanation 59:
Severe abdominal pain, distention, and absent bowel sounds are suggestive of an ileus, which is a disruption in the normal bowel motility.

Question 60:
You are assessing a patient who is unconscious and not breathing. What is the initial action you should take?

A) Begin CPR with chest compressions.
B) Administer high-flow oxygen.
C) Check for a carotid pulse.
D) Clear the airway with a finger sweep.

Answer 60:
A) Begin CPR with chest compressions.

Explanation 60:
For an unconscious, non-breathing patient, the initial action is to begin CPR with chest compressions to circulate oxygenated blood.

Question 61:
A patient with a laceration on their hand is experiencing mild bleeding. What is the appropriate method for wound care?

A) Apply a tourniquet proximal to the injury.
B) Irrigate the wound with hydrogen peroxide.
C) Apply direct pressure with a sterile dressing.
D) Leave the wound uncovered.

Answer 61:
C) Apply direct pressure with a sterile dressing.

Explanation 61:
For a mild bleeding laceration, the appropriate method is to apply direct pressure with a sterile dressing.

Question 62:
A patient with a known opioid addiction is unresponsive and not breathing. What is the initial action you should take?

A) Administer naloxone.
B) Provide intravenous glucose.
C) Perform abdominal thrusts.
D) Administer albuterol.

Answer 62:
A) Administer naloxone.

Explanation 62:
For an unresponsive, non-breathing patient with a known opioid addiction, the initial action is to administer naloxone to reverse the opioid overdose.

Question 63:
A patient presents with chest pain, diaphoresis, and pain radiating to the left arm and jaw. What condition should you suspect?

A) Pulmonary embolism
B) Myocardial infarction
C) Panic attack
D) Gastroesophageal reflux disease (GERD)

Answer 63:
B) Myocardial infarction

Explanation 63:
Chest pain, diaphoresis, and pain radiating to the left arm and jaw are classic symptoms of a myocardial infarction.

Question 64:
You are assessing a patient with a suspected spinal injury. What is the appropriate method for opening the patient's airway?

A) Tilt the patient's head backward.
B) Perform a chin lift.
C) Use a nasopharyngeal airway.
D) Administer oxygen at a high flow rate.

Answer 64:
B) Perform a chin lift.

Explanation 64:
For a patient with a suspected spinal injury, the appropriate method for opening the airway is to perform a chin lift without hyperextending the neck.

Question 65:
A patient presents with wheezing, dyspnea, and a history of allergies. What condition should you suspect?

A) Pneumothorax
B) Asthma
C) Chronic obstructive pulmonary disease (COPD)
D) Myocardial infarction

Answer 65:
B) Asthma

Explanation 65:
Wheezing, dyspnea, and a history of allergies are indicative of an asthma exacerbation.

Question 66:
You are treating a patient with a suspected pelvic fracture. What is the appropriate method for immobilizing the pelvis?

A) Place the patient in a Trendelenburg position.
B) Apply a cervical collar.
C) Use a pelvic binder or sheet.
D) Administer analgesics for pain.

Answer 66:
C) Use a pelvic binder or sheet.

Explanation 66:
For a suspected pelvic fracture, the appropriate method is to use a pelvic binder or sheet to immobilize the pelvis.

Question 67:
A patient with a history of hypertension is experiencing a severe headache, nosebleed, and altered mental status. What condition should you suspect?

A) Hypoglycemia
B) Hemorrhagic stroke
C) Tension headache
D) Seizure

Answer 67:
B) Hemorrhagic stroke

Explanation 67:
A severe headache, nosebleed, and altered mental status are concerning symptoms of a hemorrhagic stroke, especially in a patient with hypertension.

Question 68:
You are treating a patient with a suspected ankle sprain. What is the appropriate method for immobilizing the injury?

A) Apply a rigid splint.
B) Elevate the ankle.
C) Use a compression bandage.
D) Administer pain medication.

Answer 68:
A) Apply a rigid splint.

Explanation 68:
For a suspected ankle sprain, the appropriate method is to apply a rigid splint to immobilize the injury.

Question 69:
A patient with a history of seizures is experiencing uncontrolled muscle contractions and a loss of consciousness. What condition should you suspect?

A) Hypoglycemia
B) Migraine
C) Seizure
D) Stroke

Answer 69:
C) Seizure

Explanation 69:
Uncontrolled muscle contractions and a loss of consciousness are indicative of a seizure, especially in a patient with a history of seizures.

Question 70:
A patient with difficulty breathing, cyanosis, and altered mental status is likely experiencing what condition?

A) Hyperglycemia (diabetic ketoacidosis)
B) Hypoglycemia
C) Respiratory failure

D) Anxiety attack

Answer 70:
C) Respiratory failure

Explanation 70:
Difficulty breathing, cyanosis, and altered mental status are signs of respiratory failure, which can result from various causes.

Question 71:
You are treating a patient with a suspected ankle fracture. What is the appropriate method for elevating the injured leg?

A) Elevate the foot higher than the head.
B) Elevate the ankle above the level of the heart.
C) Place the leg in a dependent position.
D) Use pillows to support the leg.

Answer 71:
B) Elevate the ankle above the level of the heart.

Explanation 71:
To reduce swelling in a patient with a suspected ankle fracture, elevate the ankle above the level of the heart.

Question 72:
A patient with a history of atrial fibrillation is experiencing chest pain and shortness of breath. What is the likely diagnosis?

A) Acute myocardial infarction
B) Hyperventilation
C) Exacerbation of atrial fibrillation
D) Tension pneumothorax

Answer 72:
A) Acute myocardial infarction

Explanation 72:
In a patient with a history of atrial fibrillation experiencing chest pain and shortness of breath, the concern is an acute myocardial infarction.

Question 73:
You are assessing a patient with an altered mental status, slow heart rate, and pinpoint pupils. What medication should you consider administering?

A) Atropine
B) Epinephrine
C) Naloxone
D) Glucose

Answer 73:
A) Atropine

Explanation 73:
An altered mental status, slow heart rate, and pinpoint pupils are suggestive of a cholinergic overdose, and atropine is an appropriate treatment.

Question 74:
A patient presents with a dislocated shoulder. What is the appropriate method for immobilizing the injury?

A) Apply a rigid splint.
B) Use a sling and swathe.
C) Administer muscle relaxants.
D) Elevate the arm.

Answer 74:
B) Use a sling and swathe.

Explanation 74:
For a dislocated shoulder, the appropriate method is to use a sling and swathe to immobilize the injury.

Question 75:
A patient with a history of stroke presents with sudden-onset confusion, difficulty speaking, and weakness on one side of their body. What type of stroke should you suspect?

A) Ischemic stroke
B) Hemorrhagic stroke
C) Transient ischemic attack (TIA)
D) Migraine

Answer 75:
A) Ischemic stroke

Explanation 75:
Sudden-onset confusion, difficulty speaking, and weakness on one side of the body are typical symptoms of an ischemic stroke, which results from a blood clot.

Question 76:
You are treating a patient with a suspected femur fracture. What is the appropriate method for immobilizing the injury?

A) Apply a rigid splint.
B) Elevate the leg.
C) Use a compression bandage.
D) Administer pain medication.

Answer 76:
A) Apply a rigid splint.

Explanation 76:
For a suspected femur fracture, the appropriate method is to apply a rigid splint to immobilize the injury.

Question 77:

A patient with a known history of asthma is experiencing sudden-onset wheezing and shortness of breath. What is the appropriate treatment?

A) Administer activated charcoal.
B) Administer nitroglycerin.
C) Administer albuterol via nebulizer.
D) Apply a tourniquet to the arm.

Answer 77:
C) Administer albuterol via nebulizer.

Explanation 77:
For a patient with known asthma experiencing wheezing and shortness of breath, the appropriate treatment is albuterol via nebulizer to relieve airway constriction.

Question 78:

A patient with a known history of hypertension is experiencing a severe headache, nausea, and vomiting. What condition should you suspect?

A) Migraine
B) Tension headache
C) Hemorrhagic stroke
D) Hypertensive crisis

Answer 78:
D) Hypertensive crisis

Explanation 78:
A severe headache, nausea, and vomiting in a patient with a history of hypertension may indicate a hypertensive crisis.

Question 79:
You are treating a patient with a suspected wrist fracture. What is the appropriate method for immobilizing the injury?

A) Apply a rigid splint.
B) Elevate the wrist.
C) Use a compression bandage.
D) Administer pain medication.

Answer 79:
A) Apply a rigid splint.

Explanation 79:
For a suspected wrist fracture, the appropriate method is to apply a rigid splint to immobilize the injury.

Question 80:
A patient presents with confusion, nausea, and vomiting after consuming a large amount of alcohol. What is the likely diagnosis?

A) Alcohol poisoning
B) Gastroenteritis
C) Hypoglycemia
D) Dehydration

Answer 80:
A) Alcohol poisoning

Explanation 80:
Confusion, nausea, and vomiting after consuming a large amount of alcohol are indicative of alcohol poisoning.

Question 81:
You are assessing a patient with a suspected spinal injury. What is the appropriate method for maintaining an open airway?

A) Apply a nasopharyngeal airway.
B) Use a chin lift or jaw thrust.
C) Administer high-flow oxygen.
D) Elevate the patient's head.

Answer 81:
B) Use a chin lift or jaw thrust.

Explanation 81:
For a patient with a suspected spinal injury, it is appropriate to use a chin lift or jaw thrust to maintain an open airway without hyperextending the neck.

Question 82:
A patient presents with confusion, seizures, and a sweet, fruity odor on their breath. What condition should you suspect?

A) Hypoglycemia
B) Hyperglycemia (diabetic ketoacidosis)
C) Alcohol intoxication
D) Opioid overdose

Answer 82:
B) Hyperglycemia (diabetic ketoacidosis)

Explanation 82:
Confusion, seizures, and a sweet, fruity odor on the breath are suggestive of hyperglycemia with diabetic ketoacidosis.

Question 83:
You are treating a patient with a suspected humerus fracture. What is the appropriate method for immobilizing the injury?

A) Apply a rigid splint.
B) Elevate the arm.
C) Use a compression bandage.
D) Administer pain medication.

Answer 83:
A) Apply a rigid splint.

Explanation 83:
For a suspected humerus fracture, the appropriate method is to apply a rigid splint to immobilize the injury.

Question 84:
A patient with a history of allergies is experiencing rapid onset of swelling of the lips and tongue, hives, and difficulty breathing. What condition should you suspect?

A) Anaphylactic reaction
B) Anxiety attack
C) Asthma exacerbation
D) Heart attack

Answer 84:
A) Anaphylactic reaction

Explanation 84:
Rapid-onset swelling of the lips and tongue, hives, and difficulty breathing are classic signs of an anaphylactic reaction.

Question 85:
A patient with a history of epilepsy is experiencing confusion, involuntary muscle movements, and a bitten tongue. What is the likely diagnosis?

A) Hypoglycemia
B) Stroke
C) Seizure
D) Panic attack

Answer 85:
C) Seizure

Explanation 85:
Confusion, involuntary muscle movements, and a bitten tongue are indicative of a seizure, especially in a patient with a history of epilepsy.

Question 86:
You are treating a patient with a suspected forearm fracture. What is the appropriate method for assessing circulation?

A) Check for pupillary reaction.
B) Administer intravenous fluids.
C) Assess peripheral pulses.
D) Use a blood pressure cuff.

Answer 86:
C) Assess peripheral pulses.

Explanation 86:
To assess circulation in a patient with a suspected forearm fracture, it is appropriate to check peripheral pulses.

Question 87:
A patient with a known peanut allergy has ingested peanuts and is experiencing difficulty breathing and swelling of the face. What medication should you consider administering?

A) Aspirin
B) Nitroglycerin
C) Epinephrine
D) Albuterol

Answer 87:
C) Epinephrine

Explanation 87:
In a patient with a known peanut allergy and symptoms of difficulty breathing and facial swelling, epinephrine is the appropriate treatment.

Question 88:
A patient presents with sudden-onset chest pain that improves with rest and nitroglycerin. What condition should you suspect?

A) Myocardial infarction
B) Angina pectoris
C) Gastroesophageal reflux disease (GERD)

D) Tension headache

Answer 88:
B) Angina pectoris

Explanation 88:
Sudden-onset chest pain that improves with rest and nitroglycerin is characteristic of angina pectoris.

Question 89:
You are treating a patient with a suspected hip fracture. What is the appropriate method for immobilizing the injury?

A) Apply a rigid splint.
B) Elevate the leg.
C) Use a compression bandage.
D) Administer pain medication.

Answer 89:
A) Apply a rigid splint.

Explanation 89:
For a suspected hip fracture, the appropriate method is to apply a rigid splint to immobilize the injury.

Question 90:
A patient with a history of diabetes is experiencing confusion, rapid breathing, and fruity breath odor. What condition should you suspect?

A) Hypoglycemia
B) Hyperglycemia (diabetic ketoacidosis)
C) Alcohol intoxication
D) Anxiety attack

Answer 90:
B) Hyperglycemia (diabetic ketoacidosis)

Explanation 90:
Confusion, rapid breathing, and fruity breath odor are suggestive of hyperglycemia with diabetic ketoacidosis in a patient with diabetes.

Question 91:
You are assessing a patient with a suspected spinal injury. What is the appropriate method for maintaining the patient's airway?

A) Apply a nasopharyngeal airway.
B) Use a chin lift or jaw thrust.
C) Administer high-flow oxygen.
D) Elevate the patient's head.

Answer 91:
B) Use a chin lift or jaw thrust.

Explanation 91:
For a patient with a suspected spinal injury, it is appropriate to use a chin lift or jaw thrust to maintain an open airway without hyperextending the neck.

Question 92:
A patient with a known seizure disorder is experiencing repetitive muscle jerking and altered mental status. What is the likely diagnosis?

A) Hypoglycemia
B) Hemorrhagic stroke
C) Seizure
D) Migraine

Answer 92:
C) Seizure

Explanation 92:
Repetitive muscle jerking and altered mental status are indicative of a seizure, especially in a patient with a known seizure disorder.

Question 93:
You are treating a patient with a suspected thigh fracture. What is the appropriate method for immobilizing the injury?

A) Apply a rigid splint.
B) Elevate the leg.
C) Use a compression bandage.
D) Administer pain medication.

Answer 93:
A) Apply a rigid splint.

Explanation 93:
For a suspected thigh fracture, the appropriate method is to apply a rigid splint to immobilize the injury.

Question 94:
A patient presents with chest pain, palpitations, and dizziness. What condition should you suspect?

A) Pneumonia
B) Panic attack
C) Atrial fibrillation
D) Myocardial infarction

Answer 94:
C) Atrial fibrillation

Explanation 94:
Chest pain, palpitations, and dizziness are suggestive of atrial fibrillation, a cardiac arrhythmia.

Question 95:
You are assessing a patient with a suspected spinal injury. What is the appropriate method for immobilizing the patient?

A) Place the patient in a sitting position.
B) Apply a cervical collar.
C) Administer high-flow oxygen.
D) Keep the patient lying flat.

Answer 95:
D) Keep the patient lying flat.

Explanation 95:
For a patient with a suspected spinal injury, it is appropriate to keep the patient lying flat to prevent movement and further injury.

Question 96:
A patient with a known bee sting allergy is experiencing swelling at the site of the sting, hives, and difficulty breathing. What medication should you consider administering?

A) Aspirin
B) Nitroglycerin
C) Epinephrine
D) Albuterol

Answer 96:
C) Epinephrine

Explanation 96:
In a patient with a known bee sting allergy and symptoms of swelling, hives, and difficulty breathing, epinephrine is the appropriate treatment.

Question 97:
A patient with a history of asthma is experiencing sudden-onset wheezing and shortness of breath. What is the appropriate treatment?

A) Administer activated charcoal.
B) Administer nitroglycerin.
C) Administer albuterol via nebulizer.
D) Apply a tourniquet to the arm.

Answer 97:
C) Administer albuterol via nebulizer.

Explanation 97:
For a patient with a history of asthma experiencing sudden-onset wheezing and shortness of breath, the appropriate treatment is albuterol via nebulizer.

Question 98:
A patient presents with sudden-onset chest pain, shortness of breath, and a history of deep vein thrombosis (DVT). What condition should you suspect?

A) Pulmonary embolism
B) Myocardial infarction
C) Pneumothorax
D) Gastroesophageal reflux disease (GERD)

Answer 98:
A) Pulmonary embolism

Explanation 98:
Sudden-onset chest pain, shortness of breath, and a history of deep vein thrombosis (DVT) are concerning for a pulmonary embolism.

Question 99:
You are treating a patient with a suspected ankle sprain. What is the appropriate method for assessing the injury?

A) Perform a thorough neurological assessment.
B) Obtain a complete blood count (CBC).
C) Use diagnostic imaging such as X-rays.
D) Measure the patient's oxygen saturation.

Answer 99:
C) Use diagnostic imaging such as X-rays.

Explanation 99:
For assessing a suspected ankle sprain, diagnostic imaging, such as X-rays, can help confirm the diagnosis and rule out fractures.

Question 100:
A patient with a known history of heart failure is experiencing severe shortness of breath, frothy pink sputum, and crackles in the lungs. What is the likely diagnosis?

A) Pneumonia
B) Congestive heart failure exacerbation
C) Pulmonary embolism
D) Pneumothorax

Answer 100:
B) Congestive heart failure exacerbation

Explanation 100:
Severe shortness of breath, frothy pink sputum, and lung crackles are indicative of a congestive heart failure exacerbation in a patient with a known history of heart failure.

Question 101:
A patient is experiencing severe chest pain that worsens with deep breaths and is relieved when leaning forward. What condition should you suspect?

A) Myocardial infarction
B) Pneumothorax
C) Pericarditis
D) Anxiety attack

Answer 101:
C) Pericarditis

Explanation 101:
Chest pain worsened by deep breaths and relieved when leaning forward is characteristic of pericarditis.

Question 102:
You are treating a patient with a suspected rib fracture. What is the appropriate method for managing the injury?

A) Administer intravenous fluids.
B) Apply a rigid splint to the chest.
C) Use a compression bandage.
D) Elevate the head of the patient's bed.

Answer 102:
B) Apply a rigid splint to the chest.

Explanation 102:
For a suspected rib fracture, the appropriate method is to apply a rigid splint to the chest to minimize movement.

Question 103:
A patient with a known history of seizures is experiencing sudden jerking movements and loss of bladder control. What is the likely diagnosis?

A) Hypoglycemia
B) Hemorrhagic stroke
C) Seizure
D) Migraine

Answer 103:
C) Seizure

Explanation 103:
Sudden jerking movements and loss of bladder control are indicative of a seizure, especially in a patient with a history of seizures.

Question 104:
You are assessing a patient with a suspected spinal injury. What is the appropriate method for immobilizing the patient's head and neck?

A) Place the patient in a prone position.
B) Use a cervical collar.
C) Administer high-flow oxygen.
D) Apply a chest binder.

Answer 104:
B) Use a cervical collar.

Explanation 104:
For a patient with a suspected spinal injury, using a cervical collar is the appropriate method for immobilizing the head and neck.

Question 105:
A patient with a known bee sting allergy has been stung and is experiencing localized swelling at the sting site. What medication should you consider administering?

A) Aspirin
B) Nitroglycerin
C) Epinephrine
D) Albuterol

Answer 105:
C) Epinephrine

Explanation 105:
In a patient with a known bee sting allergy and localized swelling, epinephrine is the appropriate treatment to prevent anaphylaxis.

Question 106:
A patient with a history of chronic obstructive pulmonary disease (COPD) is experiencing severe shortness of breath, wheezing, and a chronic cough. What condition should you suspect?

A) Asthma exacerbation
B) Pneumonia
C) Heart attack
D) Emphysema

Answer 106:
A) Asthma exacerbation

Explanation 106:

Severe shortness of breath, wheezing, and a chronic cough in a patient with a history of COPD may indicate an asthma exacerbation.

Question 107:
You are treating a patient with a suspected forearm fracture. What is the appropriate method for reducing pain?

A) Apply ice to the injured area.
B) Administer intravenous fluids.
C) Elevate the arm above the level of the heart.
D) Administer analgesics.

Answer 107:
D) Administer analgesics.

Explanation 107:
To reduce pain in a patient with a suspected forearm fracture, the appropriate method is to administer analgesics.

Question 108:
A patient with a history of atrial fibrillation is experiencing chest pain, shortness of breath, and irregular pulse. What is the likely diagnosis?

A) Acute myocardial infarction
B) Hyperventilation
C) Exacerbation of atrial fibrillation
D) Tension pneumothorax

Answer 108:
A) Acute myocardial infarction

Explanation 108:
Chest pain, shortness of breath, and an irregular pulse in a patient with atrial fibrillation are concerning for an acute myocardial infarction.

Question 109:
You are treating a patient with a suspected hip fracture. What is the appropriate method for relieving pain?

A) Apply ice to the injured area.
B) Elevate the leg.
C) Administer intravenous fluids.
D) Administer analgesics.

Answer 109:
D) Administer analgesics.

Explanation 109:
To relieve pain in a patient with a suspected hip fracture, the appropriate method is to administer analgesics.

Question 110:
A patient presents with confusion, muscle weakness, and tingling in their extremities. What condition should you suspect?

A) Hypoglycemia
B) Stroke
C) Hyperkalemia
D) Anxiety attack

Answer 110:
C) Hyperkalemia

Explanation 110:
Confusion, muscle weakness, and tingling in the extremities may indicate hyperkalemia, which is an elevated level of potassium in the blood.

Question 111:
You are assessing a patient with a suspected spinal injury. What is the appropriate method for maintaining spinal alignment?

A) Perform passive range of motion exercises.
B) Apply a rigid splint to the spine.
C) Administer high-flow oxygen.
D) Keep the patient still and in a neutral position.

Answer 111:
D) Keep the patient still and in a neutral position.

Explanation 111:
For a patient with a suspected spinal injury, it is important to keep the patient still and in a neutral position to maintain spinal alignment.

Question 112:
A patient with a known history of diabetes is experiencing confusion, thirst, and frequent urination. What condition should you suspect?

A) Hypoglycemia
B) Hyperglycemia (diabetic ketoacidosis)
C) Alcohol intoxication
D) Dehydration

Answer 112:
B) Hyperglycemia (diabetic ketoacidosis)

Explanation 112:
Confusion, thirst, and frequent urination are suggestive of hyperglycemia with diabetic ketoacidosis in a patient with diabetes.

Question 113:
You are treating a patient with a suspected tibia fracture. What is the appropriate method for immobilizing the injury?

A) Apply a rigid splint.
B) Elevate the leg.
C) Use a compression bandage.
D) Administer pain medication.

Answer 113:
A) Apply a rigid splint.

Explanation 113:
For a suspected tibia fracture, the appropriate method is to apply a rigid splint to immobilize the injury.

Question 114:
A patient with a known history of allergies is experiencing red, itchy hives and facial swelling. What condition should you suspect?

A) Anaphylactic reaction
B) Anxiety attack
C) Asthma exacerbation
D) Heart attack

Answer 114:
A) Anaphylactic reaction

Explanation 114:
Red, itchy hives and facial swelling are typical signs of an anaphylactic reaction in a patient with known allergies.

Question 115:
A patient with a history of epilepsy is experiencing repetitive jerking movements and confusion. What is the likely diagnosis?

A) Hypoglycemia
B) Hemorrhagic stroke
C) Seizure
D) Panic attack

Answer 115:
C) Seizure

Explanation 115:
Repetitive jerking movements and confusion are indicative of a seizure, especially in a patient with a history of epilepsy.

Question 116:
You are treating a patient with a suspected humerus fracture. What is the appropriate method for assessing circulation in the injured arm?

A) Check for pupillary reaction.
B) Administer intravenous fluids.
C) Assess peripheral pulses.
D) Use a blood pressure cuff.

Answer 116:
C) Assess peripheral pulses.

Explanation 116:
To assess circulation in a patient with a suspected humerus fracture, it is appropriate to check peripheral pulses in the injured arm.

Question 117:
A patient with a known peanut allergy has ingested peanuts and is experiencing difficulty breathing and swelling of the face. What medication should you consider administering?

A) Aspirin
B) Nitroglycerin
C) Epinephrine
D) Albuterol

Answer 117:
C) Epinephrine

Explanation 117:
In a patient with a known peanut allergy and symptoms of difficulty breathing and facial swelling, epinephrine is the appropriate treatment.

Question 118:
A patient presents with sudden-onset chest pain, sweating, and shortness of breath. What condition should you suspect?

A) Gastroesophageal reflux disease (GERD)
B) Myocardial infarction
C) Tension headache
D) Panic attack

Answer 118:
B) Myocardial infarction

Explanation 118:
Sudden-onset chest pain, sweating, and shortness of breath are concerning symptoms of a myocardial infarction.

Question 119:
You are treating a patient with a suspected femur fracture. What is the appropriate method for immobilizing the injury?

A) Apply a rigid splint.
B) Elevate the leg.
C) Use a compression bandage.
D) Administer pain medication.

Answer 119:
A) Apply a rigid splint.

Explanation 119:
For a suspected femur fracture, the appropriate method is to apply a rigid splint to immobilize the injury.

Question 120:
A patient with a history of diabetes is experiencing confusion, rapid breathing, and fruity breath odor. What condition should you suspect?

A) Hypoglycemia
B) Hyperglycemia (diabetic ketoacidosis)
C) Alcohol intoxication
D) Anxiety attack

Answer 120:
B) Hyperglycemia (diabetic ketoacidosis)

Explanation 120:
Confusion, rapid breathing, and fruity breath odor are suggestive of hyperglycemia with diabetic ketoacidosis in a patient with diabetes.

Question 121:
You are assessing a patient with a suspected spinal injury. What is the appropriate method for maintaining spinal alignment?

A) Perform passive range of motion exercises.
B) Apply a rigid splint to the spine.
C) Administer high-flow oxygen.
D) Keep the patient still and in a neutral position.

Answer 121:
D) Keep the patient still and in a neutral position.

Explanation 121:
For a patient with a suspected spinal injury, it is important to keep the patient still and in a neutral position to maintain spinal alignment.

Question 122:
A patient with a known bee sting allergy has been stung and is experiencing localized swelling at the sting site. What medication should you consider administering?

A) Aspirin
B) Nitroglycerin
C) Epinephrine
D) Albuterol

Answer 122:
C) Epinephrine

Explanation 122:
In a patient with a known bee sting allergy and localized swelling, epinephrine is the appropriate treatment to prevent anaphylaxis.

Question 123:
A patient with a history of chronic obstructive pulmonary disease (COPD) is experiencing severe shortness of breath, wheezing, and a chronic cough. What condition should you suspect?

A) Asthma exacerbation
B) Pneumonia
C) Heart attack
D) Emphysema

Answer 123:
A) Asthma exacerbation

Explanation 123:
Severe shortness of breath, wheezing, and a chronic cough in a patient with a history of COPD may indicate an asthma exacerbation.

Question 124:
You are treating a patient with a suspected forearm fracture. What is the appropriate method for reducing pain?

A) Apply ice to the injured area.
B) Administer intravenous fluids.
C) Elevate the arm above the level of the heart.
D) Administer analgesics.

Answer 124:
D) Administer analgesics.

Explanation 124:
To reduce pain in a patient with a suspected forearm fracture, the appropriate method is to administer analgesics.

Question 125:
A patient with a known history of seizures is experiencing sudden jerking movements and loss of bladder control. What is the likely diagnosis?

A) Hypoglycemia
B) Hemorrhagic stroke
C) Seizure
D) Migraine

Answer 125:
C) Seizure

Explanation 125:
Sudden jerking movements and loss of bladder control are indicative of a seizure, especially in a patient with a history of seizures.

Question 126:
You are assessing a patient with a suspected spinal injury. What is the appropriate method for immobilizing the patient's head and neck?

A) Place the patient in a prone position.
B) Use a cervical collar.
C) Administer high-flow oxygen.
D) Apply a chest binder.

Answer 126:
B) Use a cervical collar.

Explanation 126:
For a patient with a suspected spinal injury, using a cervical collar is the appropriate method for immobilizing the head and neck.

Question 127:

A patient with a known peanut allergy has ingested peanuts and is experiencing difficulty breathing and swelling of the face. What medication should you consider administering?

A) Aspirin
B) Nitroglycerin
C) Epinephrine
D) Albuterol

Answer 127:
C) Epinephrine

Explanation 127:
In a patient with a known peanut allergy and symptoms of difficulty breathing and facial swelling, epinephrine is the appropriate treatment.

Question 128:

A patient presents with sudden-onset chest pain, sweating, and shortness of breath. What condition should you suspect?

A) Gastroesophageal reflux disease (GERD)
B) Myocardial infarction
C) Tension headache
D) Panic attack

Answer 128:
B) Myocardial infarction

Explanation 128:
Sudden-onset chest pain, sweating, and shortness of breath are concerning symptoms of a myocardial infarction.

Question 129:
You are treating a patient with a suspected femur fracture. What is the appropriate method for immobilizing the injury?

A) Apply a rigid splint.
B) Elevate the leg.
C) Use a compression bandage.
D) Administer pain medication.

Answer 129:
A) Apply a rigid splint.

Explanation 129:
For a suspected femur fracture, the appropriate method is to apply a rigid splint to immobilize the injury.

Question 130:
A patient with a history of diabetes is experiencing confusion, rapid breathing, and fruity breath odor. What condition should you suspect?

A) Hypoglycemia
B) Hyperglycemia (diabetic ketoacidosis)
C) Alcohol intoxication
D) Anxiety attack

Answer 130:
B) Hyperglycemia (diabetic ketoacidosis)

Explanation 130:
Confusion, rapid breathing, and fruity breath odor are suggestive of hyperglycemia with diabetic ketoacidosis in a patient with diabetes.

Question 131:
You are assessing a patient with a suspected spinal injury. What is the appropriate method for maintaining spinal alignment?

A) Perform passive range of motion exercises.
B) Apply a rigid splint to the spine.
C) Administer high-flow oxygen.
D) Keep the patient still and in a neutral position.

Answer 131:
D) Keep the patient still and in a neutral position.

Explanation 131:
For a patient with a suspected spinal injury, it is important to keep the patient still and in a neutral position to maintain spinal alignment.

Question 132:
A patient with a known bee sting allergy has been stung and is experiencing localized swelling at the sting site. What medication should you consider administering?

A) Aspirin
B) Nitroglycerin
C) Epinephrine
D) Albuterol

Answer 132:
C) Epinephrine

Explanation 132:
In a patient with a known bee sting allergy and localized swelling, epinephrine is the appropriate treatment to prevent anaphylaxis.

Question 133:
A patient with a history of chronic obstructive pulmonary disease (COPD) is experiencing severe shortness of breath, wheezing, and a chronic cough. What condition should you suspect?

A) Asthma exacerbation
B) Pneumonia
C) Heart attack
D) Emphysema

Answer 133:
A) Asthma exacerbation

Explanation 133:

Severe shortness of breath, wheezing, and a chronic cough in a patient with a history of COPD may indicate an asthma exacerbation.

Question 134:
You are treating a patient with a suspected forearm fracture. What is the appropriate method for reducing pain?

A) Apply ice to the injured area.
B) Administer intravenous fluids.
C) Elevate the arm above the level of the heart.
D) Administer analgesics.

Answer 134:
D) Administer analgesics.

Explanation 134:
To reduce pain in a patient with a suspected forearm fracture, the appropriate method is to administer analgesics.

Question 135:
A patient with a known history of seizures is experiencing sudden jerking movements and loss of bladder control. What is the likely diagnosis?

A) Hypoglycemia
B) Hemorrhagic stroke
C) Seizure
D) Migraine

Answer 135:
C) Seizure

Explanation 135:
Sudden jerking movements and loss of bladder control are indicative of a seizure, especially in a patient with a history of seizures.

Question 136:
You are assessing a patient with a suspected spinal injury. What is the appropriate method for immobilizing the patient's head and neck?

A) Place the patient in a prone position.
B) Use a cervical collar.
C) Administer high-flow oxygen.
D) Apply a chest binder.

Answer 136:
B) Use a cervical collar.

Explanation 136:
For a patient with a suspected spinal injury, using a cervical collar is the appropriate method for immobilizing the head and neck.

Question 137:
A patient with a known peanut allergy has ingested peanuts and is experiencing difficulty breathing and swelling of the face. What medication should you consider administering?

A) Aspirin
B) Nitroglycerin
C) Epinephrine
D) Albuterol

Answer 137:
C) Epinephrine

Explanation 137:
In a patient with a known peanut allergy and symptoms of difficulty breathing and facial swelling, epinephrine is the appropriate treatment.

Question 138:
A patient presents with sudden-onset chest pain, sweating, and shortness of breath. What condition should you suspect?

A) Gastroesophageal reflux disease (GERD)
B) Myocardial infarction
C) Tension headache
D) Panic attack

Answer 138:
B) Myocardial infarction

Explanation 138:
Sudden-onset chest pain, sweating, and shortness of breath are concerning symptoms of a myocardial infarction.

Question 139:
You are treating a patient with a suspected femur fracture. What is the appropriate method for immobilizing the injury?

A) Apply a rigid splint.
B) Elevate the leg.
C) Use a compression bandage.
D) Administer pain medication.

Answer 139:
A) Apply a rigid splint.

Explanation 139:
For a suspected femur fracture, the appropriate method is to apply a rigid splint to immobilize the injury.

Question 140:
A patient with a history of diabetes is experiencing confusion, rapid breathing, and fruity breath odor. What condition should you suspect?

A) Hypoglycemia
B) Hyperglycemia (diabetic ketoacidosis)
C) Alcohol intoxication
D) Anxiety attack

Answer 140:
B) Hyperglycemia (diabetic ketoacidosis)

Explanation 140:
Confusion, rapid breathing, and fruity breath odor are suggestive of hyperglycemia with diabetic ketoacidosis in a patient with diabetes.

Question 141:
You are assessing a patient with a suspected spinal injury. What is the appropriate method for maintaining spinal alignment?

A) Perform passive range of motion exercises.
B) Apply a rigid splint to the spine.
C) Administer high-flow oxygen.
D) Keep the patient still and in a neutral position.

Answer 141:
D) Keep the patient still and in a neutral position.

Explanation 141:
For a patient with a suspected spinal injury, it is important to keep the patient still and in a neutral position to maintain spinal alignment.

Question 142:
A patient with a known bee sting allergy has been stung and is experiencing localized swelling at the sting site. What medication should you consider administering?

A) Aspirin
B) Nitroglycerin
C) Epinephrine
D) Albuterol

Answer 142:
C) Epinephrine

Explanation 142:
In a patient with a known bee sting allergy and localized swelling, epinephrine is the appropriate treatment to prevent anaphylaxis.

Question 143:
A patient with a history of chronic obstructive pulmonary disease (COPD) is experiencing severe shortness of breath, wheezing, and a chronic cough. What condition should you suspect?

A) Asthma exacerbation
B) Pneumonia
C) Heart attack
D) Emphysema

Answer 143:
A) Asthma exacerbation

Explanation 143:
Severe shortness of breath, wheezing, and a chronic cough in a patient with a history of COPD may indicate an asthma exacerbation.

Question 144:
You are treating a patient with a suspected forearm fracture. What is the appropriate method for reducing pain?

A) Apply ice to the injured area.
B) Administer intravenous fluids.
C) Elevate the arm above the level of the heart.
D) Administer analgesics.

Answer 144:
D) Administer analgesics.

Explanation 144:
To reduce pain in a patient with a suspected forearm fracture, the appropriate method is to administer analgesics.

Question 145:
A patient with a history of epilepsy is experiencing sudden jerking movements and loss of bladder control. What is the likely diagnosis?

A) Hypoglycemia
B) Hemorrhagic stroke
C) Seizure
D) Migraine

Answer 145:
C) Seizure

Explanation 145:
Sudden jerking movements and loss of bladder control are indicative of a seizure, especially in a patient with a history of epilepsy.

Question 146:
You are assessing a patient with a suspected spinal injury. What is the appropriate method for immobilizing the patient's head and neck?

A) Place the patient in a prone position.
B) Use a cervical collar.
C) Administer high-flow oxygen.
D) Apply a chest binder.

Answer 146:
B) Use a cervical collar.

Explanation 146:
For a patient with a suspected spinal injury, using a cervical collar is the appropriate method for immobilizing the head and neck.

Question 147:
A patient with a known peanut allergy has ingested peanuts and is experiencing difficulty breathing and swelling of the face. What medication should you consider administering?

A) Aspirin
B) Nitroglycerin
C) Epinephrine

D) Albuterol

Answer 147:
C) Epinephrine

Explanation 147:
In a patient with a known peanut allergy and symptoms of difficulty breathing and facial swelling, epinephrine is the appropriate treatment to prevent anaphylaxis.

Question 148:
A patient presents with sudden-onset chest pain, sweating, and shortness of breath. What condition should you suspect?

A) Gastroesophageal reflux disease (GERD)
B) Myocardial infarction
C) Tension headache
D) Panic attack

Answer 148:
B) Myocardial infarction

Explanation 148:
Sudden-onset chest pain, sweating, and shortness of breath are concerning symptoms of a myocardial infarction.

Question 149:
You are treating a patient with a suspected femur fracture. What is the appropriate method for immobilizing the injury?

A) Apply a rigid splint.
B) Elevate the leg.
C) Use a compression bandage.
D) Administer pain medication.

Answer 149:
A) Apply a rigid splint.

Explanation 149:

For a suspected femur fracture, the appropriate method is to apply a rigid splint to immobilize the injury.

Question 150:
A patient with a history of diabetes is experiencing confusion, rapid breathing, and fruity breath odor. What condition should you suspect?

A) Hypoglycemia
B) Hyperglycemia (diabetic ketoacidosis)
C) Alcohol intoxication
D) Anxiety attack

Answer 150:
B) Hyperglycemia (diabetic ketoacidosis)

Explanation 150:
Confusion, rapid breathing, and fruity breath odor are suggestive of hyperglycemia with diabetic ketoacidosis in a patient with diabetes.

Question 151:
You are assessing a patient with a suspected spinal injury. What is the appropriate method for maintaining spinal alignment?

A) Perform passive range of motion exercises.
B) Apply a rigid splint to the spine.
C) Administer high-flow oxygen.
D) Keep the patient still and in a neutral position.

Answer 151:
D) Keep the patient still and in a neutral position.

Explanation 151:
For a patient with a suspected spinal injury, it is important to keep the patient still and in a neutral position to maintain spinal alignment.

Question 152:
A patient with a known bee sting allergy has been stung and is experiencing localized swelling at the sting site. What medication should you consider administering?

A) Aspirin
B) Nitroglycerin
C) Epinephrine
D) Albuterol

Answer 152:
C) Epinephrine

Explanation 152:
In a patient with a known bee sting allergy and localized swelling, epinephrine is the appropriate treatment to prevent anaphylaxis.

Question 153:
A patient with a history of chronic obstructive pulmonary disease (COPD) is experiencing severe shortness of breath, wheezing, and a chronic cough. What condition should you suspect?

A) Asthma exacerbation
B) Pneumonia
C) Heart attack
D) Emphysema

Answer 153:
A) Asthma exacerbation

Explanation 153:
Severe shortness of breath, wheezing, and a chronic cough in a patient with a history of COPD may indicate an asthma exacerbation.

Question 154:
You are treating a patient with a suspected forearm fracture. What is the appropriate method for reducing pain?

A) Apply ice to the injured area.
B) Administer intravenous fluids.
C) Elevate the arm above the level of the heart.
D) Administer analgesics.

Answer 154:
D) Administer analgesics.

Explanation 154:
To reduce pain in a patient with a suspected forearm fracture, the appropriate method is to administer analgesics.

Question 155:
A patient with a known history of seizures is experiencing sudden jerking movements and loss of bladder control. What is the likely diagnosis?

A) Hypoglycemia
B) Hemorrhagic stroke
C) Seizure
D) Migraine

Answer 155:
C) Seizure

Explanation 155:
Sudden jerking movements and loss of bladder control are indicative of a seizure, especially in a patient with a history of seizures.

Question 156:
You are assessing a patient with a suspected spinal injury. What is the appropriate method for immobilizing the patient's head and neck?

A) Place the patient in a prone position.
B) Use a cervical collar.
C) Administer high-flow oxygen.
D) Apply a chest binder.

Answer 156:
B) Use a cervical collar.

Explanation 156:
For a patient with a suspected spinal injury, using a cervical collar is the appropriate method for immobilizing the head and neck.

Question 157:
A patient with a known peanut allergy has ingested peanuts and is experiencing difficulty breathing and swelling of the face. What medication should you consider administering?

A) Aspirin
B) Nitroglycerin
C) Epinephrine
D) Albuterol

Answer 157:
C) Epinephrine

Explanation 157:
In a patient with a known peanut allergy and symptoms of difficulty breathing and facial swelling, epinephrine is the appropriate treatment to prevent anaphylaxis.

Question 158:
A patient presents with sudden-onset chest pain, sweating, and shortness of breath. What condition should you suspect?

A) Gastroesophageal reflux disease (GERD)
B) Myocardial infarction
C) Tension headache
D) Panic attack

Answer 158:
B) Myocardial infarction

Explanation 158:

Sudden-onset chest pain, sweating, and shortness of breath are concerning symptoms of a myocardial infarction.

Question 159:
You are treating a patient with a suspected femur fracture. What is the appropriate method for immobilizing the injury?

A) Apply a rigid splint.
B) Elevate the leg.
C) Use a compression bandage.
D) Administer pain medication.

Answer 159:
A) Apply a rigid splint.

Explanation 159:
For a suspected femur fracture, the appropriate method is to apply a rigid splint to immobilize the injury.

Question 160:
A patient with a history of diabetes is experiencing confusion, rapid breathing, and fruity breath odor. What condition should you suspect?

A) Hypoglycemia
B) Hyperglycemia (diabetic ketoacidosis)
C) Alcohol intoxication
D) Anxiety attack

Answer 160:
B) Hyperglycemia (diabetic ketoacidosis)

Explanation 160:
Confusion, rapid breathing, and fruity breath odor are suggestive of hyperglycemia with diabetic ketoacidosis in a patient with diabetes.

Question 161:
You are assessing a patient with a suspected spinal injury. What is the appropriate method for maintaining spinal alignment?

A) Perform passive range of motion exercises.
B) Apply a rigid splint to the spine.
C) Administer high-flow oxygen.
D) Keep the patient still and in a neutral position.

Answer 161:
D) Keep the patient still and in a neutral position.

Explanation 161:
For a patient with a suspected spinal injury, it is important to keep the patient still and in a neutral position to maintain spinal alignment.

Question 162:
A patient with a known bee sting allergy has been stung and is experiencing localized swelling at the sting site. What medication should you consider administering?

A) Aspirin
B) Nitroglycerin
C) Epinephrine
D) Albuterol

Answer 162:
C) Epinephrine

Explanation 162:
In a patient with a known bee sting allergy and localized swelling, epinephrine is the appropriate treatment to prevent anaphylaxis.

Question 163:
A patient with a history of chronic obstructive pulmonary disease (COPD) is experiencing severe shortness of breath, wheezing, and a chronic cough. What condition should you suspect?

A) Asthma exacerbation
B) Pneumonia
C) Heart attack
D) Emphysema

Answer 163:
A) Asthma exacerbation

Explanation 163:
Severe shortness of breath, wheezing, and a chronic cough in a patient with a history of COPD may indicate an asthma exacerbation.

Question 164:
You are treating a patient with a suspected forearm fracture. What is the appropriate method for reducing pain?

A) Apply ice to the injured area.
B) Administer intravenous fluids.
C) Elevate the arm above the level of the heart.
D) Administer analgesics.

Answer 164:
D) Administer analgesics.

Explanation 164:
To reduce pain in a patient with a suspected forearm fracture, the appropriate method is to administer analgesics.

Question 165:
A patient with a known history of seizures is experiencing sudden jerking movements and loss of bladder control. What is the likely diagnosis?

A) Hypoglycemia
B) Hemorrhagic stroke
C) Seizure
D) Migraine

Answer 165:
C) Seizure

Explanation 165:
Sudden jerking movements and loss of bladder control are indicative of a seizure, especially in a patient with a history of seizures.

Question 166:
You are assessing a patient with a suspected spinal injury. What is the appropriate method for immobilizing the patient's head and neck?

A) Place the patient in a prone position.
B) Use a cervical collar.
C) Administer high-flow oxygen.
D) Apply a chest binder.

Answer 166:
B) Use a cervical collar.

Explanation 166:
For a patient with a suspected spinal injury, using a cervical collar is the appropriate method for immobilizing the head and neck.

Question 167:
A patient with a known peanut allergy has ingested peanuts and is experiencing difficulty breathing and swelling of the face. What medication should you consider administering?

A) Aspirin
B) Nitroglycerin
C) Epinephrine
D) Albuterol

Answer 167:
C) Epinephrine

Explanation 167:
In a patient with a known peanut allergy and symptoms of difficulty breathing and facial swelling, epinephrine is the appropriate treatment to prevent anaphylaxis.

Question 168:
A patient presents with sudden-onset chest pain, sweating, and shortness of breath. What condition should you suspect?

A) Gastroesophageal reflux disease (GERD)
B) Myocardial infarction
C) Tension headache
D) Panic attack

Answer 168:
B) Myocardial infarction

Explanation 168:
Sudden-onset chest pain, sweating, and shortness of breath are concerning symptoms of a myocardial infarction.

Question 169:
You are treating a patient with a suspected femur fracture. What is the appropriate method for immobilizing the injury?

A) Apply a rigid splint.
B) Elevate the leg.
C) Use a compression bandage.
D) Administer pain medication.

Answer 169:
A) Apply a rigid splint.

Explanation 169:
For a suspected femur fracture, the appropriate method is to apply a rigid splint to immobilize the injury.

Question 170:
A patient with a history of diabetes is experiencing confusion, rapid breathing, and fruity breath odor. What condition should you suspect?

A) Hypoglycemia
B) Hyperglycemia (diabetic ketoacidosis)
C) Alcohol intoxication
D) Anxiety attack

Answer 170:
B) Hyperglycemia (diabetic ketoacidosis)

Explanation 170:
Confusion, rapid breathing, and fruity breath odor are suggestive of hyperglycemia with diabetic ketoacidosis in a patient with diabetes.

Question 171:
A patient with a history of hypertension complains of a severe headache, confusion, and visual disturbances. What condition should you suspect?

A) Hypoglycemia
B) Stroke
C) Migraine
D) Anxiety attack

Answer 171:
B) Stroke

Explanation 171:
A severe headache, confusion, and visual disturbances in a patient with a history of hypertension are concerning symptoms of a stroke.

Question 172:
You are assessing a patient with a suspected ankle fracture. What is the appropriate method for reducing pain?

A) Apply ice to the injured area.
B) Administer intravenous fluids.
C) Elevate the leg.
D) Administer analgesics.

Answer 172:
D) Administer analgesics.

Explanation 172:
To reduce pain in a patient with a suspected ankle fracture, the appropriate method is to administer analgesics.

Question 173:
A patient with a history of asthma is experiencing difficulty breathing, wheezing, and a persistent cough. What condition should you suspect?

A) Bronchitis
B) Pneumonia
C) Asthma exacerbation
D) Heart attack

Answer 173:
C) Asthma exacerbation

Explanation 173:
Difficulty breathing, wheezing, and a persistent cough in a patient with a history of asthma may indicate an asthma exacerbation.

Question 174:
You are treating a patient with a suspected wrist fracture. What is the appropriate method for immobilizing the injury?

A) Apply ice to the injured area.
B) Elevate the wrist above the level of the heart.
C) Use a compression bandage.
D) Apply a splint.

Answer 174:
D) Apply a splint.

Explanation 174:
For a suspected wrist fracture, the appropriate method is to apply a splint to immobilize the injury.

Question 175:
A patient with a known bee sting allergy has been stung and is experiencing generalized itching, hives, and difficulty breathing. What medication should you consider administering?

A) Aspirin
B) Nitroglycerin
C) Epinephrine
D) Albuterol

Answer 175:
C) Epinephrine

Explanation 175:

In a patient with a known bee sting allergy and symptoms of generalized itching, hives, and difficulty breathing, epinephrine is the appropriate treatment to prevent anaphylaxis.

Question 176:
A patient with a history of diabetes is experiencing confusion, rapid breathing, and a fruity breath odor. What condition should you suspect?

A) Hypoglycemia
B) Hyperglycemia (diabetic ketoacidosis)
C) Alcohol intoxication
D) Anxiety attack

Answer 176:
B) Hyperglycemia (diabetic ketoacidosis)

Explanation 176:
Confusion, rapid breathing, and a fruity breath odor are suggestive of hyperglycemia with diabetic ketoacidosis in a patient with diabetes.

Question 177:
You are assessing a patient with a suspected hip fracture. What is the appropriate method for immobilizing the injury?

A) Apply ice to the injured area.
B) Elevate the leg.
C) Use a compression bandage.
D) Apply a splint.

Answer 177:
D) Apply a splint.

Explanation 177:
For a suspected hip fracture, the appropriate method is to apply a splint to immobilize the injury.

Question 178:
A patient with a known peanut allergy has ingested peanuts and is experiencing difficulty breathing and swelling of the face. What medication should you consider administering?

A) Aspirin
B) Nitroglycerin
C) Epinephrine
D) Albuterol

Answer 178:
C) Epinephrine

Explanation 178:
In a patient with a known peanut allergy and symptoms of difficulty breathing and facial swelling, epinephrine is the appropriate treatment to prevent anaphylaxis.

Question 179:
A patient presents with sudden-onset chest pain, sweating, and shortness of breath. What condition should you suspect?

A) Gastroesophageal reflux disease (GERD)
B) Myocardial infarction
C) Tension headache
D) Panic attack

Answer 179:
B) Myocardial infarction

Explanation 179:
Sudden-onset chest pain, sweating, and shortness of breath are concerning symptoms of a myocardial infarction.

Question 180:
You are treating a patient with a suspected radius and ulna fracture. What is the appropriate method for immobilizing the injury?

A) Apply ice to the injured area.
B) Elevate the arm above the level of the heart.
C) Use a compression bandage.
D) Apply a splint.

Answer 180:
D) Apply a splint.

Explanation 180:
For a suspected radius and ulna fracture, the appropriate method is to apply a splint to immobilize the injury.

Question 181:
A patient with a history of epilepsy is experiencing sudden jerking movements and loss of bladder control. What is the likely diagnosis?

A) Hypoglycemia
B) Hemorrhagic stroke
C) Seizure
D) Migraine

Answer 181:
C) Seizure

Explanation 181:
Sudden jerking movements and loss of bladder control are indicative of a seizure, especially in a patient with a history of epilepsy.

Question 182:
You are assessing a patient with a suspected spinal injury. What is the appropriate method for immobilizing the patient's head and neck?

A) Place the patient in a prone position.
B) Use a cervical collar.
C) Administer high-flow oxygen.
D) Apply a chest binder.

Answer 182:
B) Use a cervical collar.

Explanation 182:
For a patient with a suspected spinal injury, using a cervical collar is the appropriate method for immobilizing the head and neck.

Question 183:
A patient with a known bee sting allergy has been stung and is experiencing localized swelling at the sting site. What medication should you consider administering?

A) Aspirin
B) Nitroglycerin
C) Epinephrine
D) Albuterol

Answer 183:
C) Epinephrine

Explanation 183:
In a patient with a known bee sting allergy and localized swelling, epinephrine is the appropriate treatment to prevent anaphylaxis.

Question 184:
A patient with a history of chronic obstructive pulmonary disease (COPD) is experiencing severe shortness of breath, wheezing, and a chronic cough. What condition should you suspect?

A) Asthma exacerbation
B) Pneumonia
C) Heart attack
D) Emphysema

Answer 184:
A) Asthma exacerbation

Explanation 184:

Severe shortness of breath, wheezing, and a chronic cough in a patient with a history of COPD may indicate an asthma exacerbation.

Question 185:
You are treating a patient with a suspected ankle fracture. What is the appropriate method for reducing pain?

A) Apply ice to the injured area.
B) Administer intravenous fluids.
C) Elevate the leg.
D) Administer analgesics.

Answer 185:
D) Administer analgesics.

Explanation 185:
To reduce pain in a patient with a suspected ankle fracture, the appropriate method is to administer analgesics.

Question 186:
A patient with a history of hypertension complains of a severe headache, confusion, and visual disturbances. What condition should you suspect?

A) Hypoglycemia
B) Stroke
C) Migraine
D) Anxiety attack

Answer 186:
B) Stroke

Explanation 186:
A severe headache, confusion, and visual disturbances in a patient with a history of hypertension are concerning symptoms of a stroke.

Question 187:
You are assessing a patient with a suspected ankle fracture. What is the appropriate method for immobilizing the injury?

A) Apply ice to the injured area.
B) Elevate the leg.
C) Use a compression bandage.
D) Apply a splint.

Answer 187:
D) Apply a splint.

Explanation 187:
For a suspected ankle fracture, the appropriate method is to apply a splint to immobilize the injury.

Question 188:
A patient with a history of asthma is experiencing difficulty breathing, wheezing, and a persistent cough. What condition should you suspect?

A) Bronchitis
B) Pneumonia
C) Asthma exacerbation
D) Heart attack

Answer 188:
C) Asthma exacerbation

Explanation 188:
Difficulty breathing, wheezing, and a persistent cough in a patient with a history of asthma may indicate an asthma exacerbation.

Question 189:
You are treating a patient with a suspected wrist fracture. What is the appropriate method for immobilizing the injury?

A) Apply ice to the injured area.
B) Elevate the wrist above the level of the heart.
C) Use a compression bandage.
D) Apply a splint.

Answer 189:
D) Apply a splint.

Explanation 189:
For a suspected wrist fracture, the appropriate method is to apply a splint to immobilize the injury.

Question 190:
A patient with a known bee sting allergy has been stung and is experiencing generalized itching, hives, and difficulty breathing. What medication should you consider administering?

A) Aspirin
B) Nitroglycerin
C) Epinephrine
D) Albuterol

Answer 190:
C) Epinephrine

Explanation 190:
In a patient with a known bee sting allergy and symptoms of generalized itching, hives, and difficulty breathing, epinephrine is the appropriate treatment to prevent anaphylaxis.

Question 191:
A patient with a history of diabetes is experiencing confusion, rapid breathing, and a fruity breath odor. What condition should you suspect?

A) Hypoglycemia
B) Hyperglycemia (diabetic ketoacidosis)
C) Alcohol intoxication
D) Anxiety attack

Answer 191:
B) Hyperglycemia (diabetic ketoacidosis)

Explanation 191:

Confusion, rapid breathing, and a fruity breath odor are suggestive of hyperglycemia with diabetic ketoacidosis in a patient with diabetes.

Question 192:
You are assessing a patient with a suspected hip fracture. What is the appropriate method for immobilizing the injury?

A) Apply ice to the injured area.
B) Elevate the leg.
C) Use a compression bandage.
D) Apply a splint.

Answer 192:
D) Apply a splint.

Explanation 192:
For a suspected hip fracture, the appropriate method is to apply a splint to immobilize the injury.

Question 193:
A patient with a known peanut allergy has ingested peanuts and is experiencing difficulty breathing and swelling of the face. What medication should you consider administering?

A) Aspirin
B) Nitroglycerin
C) Epinephrine
D) Albuterol

Answer 193:
C) Epinephrine

Explanation 193:
In a patient with a known peanut allergy and symptoms of difficulty breathing and facial swelling, epinephrine is the appropriate treatment to prevent anaphylaxis.

Question 194:
A patient presents with sudden-onset chest pain, sweating, and shortness of breath. What condition should you suspect?

A) Gastroesophageal reflux disease (GERD)
B) Myocardial infarction
C) Tension headache
D) Panic attack

Answer 194:
B) Myocardial infarction

Explanation 194:
Sudden-onset chest pain, sweating, and shortness of breath are concerning symptoms of a myocardial infarction.

Question 195:
You are treating a patient with a suspected radius and ulna fracture. What is the appropriate method for reducing pain?

A) Apply ice to the injured area.
B) Administer intravenous fluids.
C) Elevate the arm above the level of the heart.
D) Administer analgesics.

Answer 195:
D) Administer analgesics.

Explanation 195:
To reduce pain in a patient with a suspected radius and ulna fracture, the appropriate method is to administer analgesics.

Question 196:
A patient with a history of epilepsy is experiencing sudden jerking movements and loss of bladder control. What is the likely diagnosis?

A) Hypoglycemia
B) Hemorrhagic stroke
C) Seizure
D) Migraine

Answer 196:
C) Seizure

Explanation 196:
Sudden jerking movements and loss of bladder control are indicative of a seizure, especially in a patient with a history of epilepsy.

Question 197:
You are assessing a patient with a suspected spinal injury. What is the appropriate method for immobilizing the patient's head and neck?

A) Place the patient in a prone position.
B) Use a cervical collar.
C) Administer high-flow oxygen.
D) Apply a chest binder.

Answer 197:
B) Use a cervical collar.

Explanation 197:
For a patient with a suspected spinal injury, using a cervical collar is the appropriate method for immobilizing the head and neck.

Question 198:
A patient with a known bee sting allergy has been stung and is experiencing localized swelling at the sting site. What medication should you consider administering?

A) Aspirin
B) Nitroglycerin
C) Epinephrine
D) Albuterol

Answer 198:
C) Epinephrine

Explanation 198:
In a patient with a known bee sting allergy and localized swelling, epinephrine is the appropriate treatment to prevent anaphylaxis.

Question 199:
A patient with a history of chronic obstructive pulmonary disease (COPD) is experiencing severe shortness of breath, wheezing, and a chronic cough. What condition should you suspect?

A) Asthma exacerbation
B) Pneumonia
C) Heart attack
D) Emphysema

Answer 199:
A) Asthma exacerbation

Explanation 199:
Severe shortness of breath, wheezing, and a chronic cough in a patient with a history of COPD may indicate an asthma exacerbation.

Question 200:
You are treating a patient with a suspected ankle fracture. What is the appropriate method for immobilizing the injury?

A) Apply ice to the injured area.
B) Administer intravenous fluids.
C) Elevate the leg.
D) Apply a splint.

Answer 200:
D) Apply a splint.

Explanation 200:
For a suspected ankle fracture, the appropriate method is to apply a splint to immobilize the injury.